# *THE* Younger Next Year® Back Book

The Whole-Body Plan to Conquer Back Pain Forever

Chris Crowley &
Jeremy James, DC, CSCS

WORKMAN PUBLISHING • NEW YORK

YOUNGER NEXT YEAR is a registered trademark of Christopher Crowley and
Henry S. Lodge

Design by Galen Smith
Additional illustrations by James Williamson

Library of Congress Cataloging-in-Publication Data is available.

Paperback ISBN 978-1-5235-0447-3
Hardcover ISBN 978-1-5235-0296-7

Workman books are available at special discounts when purchased in bulk for
premiums and sales promotions as well as for fund-raising or educational use.
Special editions or book excerpts can also be created to specification. For details,
contact the Special Sales Director at the address below, or send an email to
specialmarkets@workman.com.

Workman Publishing Co., Inc.
225 Varick Street
New York, NY 10014
workman.com
youngernextyear.com

Printed in the United States of America
First printing August 2018
10 9 8 7 6 5 4 3 2 1

The program of exercise in *The Younger Next Year Back Book* is safe and
scientifically structured. Nevertheless, consult your doctor before beginning this
or any exercise program—particularly if you have ever had a heart attack or been
diagnosed with cardiovascular or coronary heart disease; have frequent chest pains
or often feel faint or dizzy upon physical exertion; have high blood pressure or high
cholesterol levels, diabetes, or liver or kidney disease; are female and more than
three months pregnant or less than three months postpartum; or are under eighteen
years of age. In addition, ask your doctor's advice if you have muscle, joint, or bone
problems that might be aggravated by exercise. And for Pete's sake, if you don't feel
well or if something hurts, stop.

# Contents

# Introduction

When Chris Crowley first walked into my office eight years ago seeking my professional advice for his nagging hip, little did I know that we would soon embark on a friendship and working relationship that would have such an impact on so many people. Having spent the last three decades of my career in the health and fitness industry, I had heard about Chris, the renowned author of the *New York Times* bestselling Younger Next Year (YNY) books. After working with him for several months it was a humbling surprise when he asked me to contribute to the Younger Next Year sequels including *Thinner This Year* and *Younger Next Year: The Exercise Program*. Now with over 2 million copies of the YNY series in print worldwide, I am still awed by the many testimonials we receive from those whose lives have been positively changed by these books. If this is your first YNY book, you are in for a treat. Chris has a gift for taking complicated medical concepts and bringing them to life with a fun, imaginative, and practical touch. Chris performs his magic once again in the *Younger Next Year Back Book*.

This time Chris brings on board the brilliance of Jeremy James, DC, CSCS.

I have had the privilege of working with Jeremy James here in Aspen for several years. Jeremy is a superb clinician, who, while he comes from a chiropractic background, does not limit his treatment approach to a single professional viewpoint. His primary objective is to provide his patients and clients with the most resourceful information that will improve their health, and he is willing to push the boundaries to do so better. Jeremy's career is defined by exploring concepts and strategies to help those who suffer from back pain. I personally know many of his patients and have heard their grateful responses, and it is very impressive. They come from all over the country to reclaim control of their lives, and with his help, the vast majority do precisely that. Jeremy's passion led to the protocol that is the basis of this remarkable book. The book is long overdue. Too many people's lives are ruled by chronic back pain.

During my long career as a physical therapist specializing in sports medicine injuries, I have had the privilege to treat thousands of patients with a variety of musculoskeletal ailments. Yet the most prevalent and disabling diagnosis is back pain. For so many patients, back pain has a crippling effect on their lifestyle, a constant grip on everything they want to do or can no longer do. Having had to overcome my own back problems (several herniated discs from decades of ice hockey, beginning at age six), I can relate to the daily difficulties that these patients endure. Who would imagine that the spine, with all of its supporting musculature and ligaments, could be so fragile? The human body is beautifully designed to express movement in all its forms and fashions, to be free and limitless in space. So what is it about the spine that makes it so vulnerable?

From a structural and evolutionary perspective, the spine is more important than any of the other sets of joints in the human body. It encloses the tubular network of nerves known as the spinal cord that together with the brain forms the central nervous system. The spinal cord is critical for daily functions, but keeping it working right is also essential for our very survival. Injure a knee or shoulder and you can still function. It may be painful and not ideal, but you can still find a way to go up stairs, lift things, and complete daily tasks. Do something serious to your spine or any of its surrounding soft tissue structures and you're facing a completely different situation. The whole body shuts down. Sometimes just getting out of bed is impossible, and the thought of sitting up and concentrating on daily activities is overwhelming. No wonder people with back pain get depressed. Despair, agony, frustration all set in as the ability to move, to play, and simply to have fun becomes severely impaired. Anyone who has experienced intense back pain can relate to the urgency of restoring spine health.

If you've tried to solve the mystery of your back pain, you know it is often a complicated road filled with doubts and questions. What type of back problem do I have? How do I fix it? How much time will it take to heal? What type of exercise should I do? Should I have surgery? Will I ever have a normal life? In this expanding world of medical treatments and professions we have choices. Many of the patients I've worked with have tried just about every treatment and exercise routine imaginable, yet they still complain of constant pain or frequent episodes of reoccurrence. They are preoccupied with their back problems and frustrated and confused as to what to do about them. If only there were a guide, a means to better understanding what to do to stop this cycle of misery, a master plan with progressions. Not simply a rehab program, but a lifestyle program. (And if you have serious back pain, you certainly do need to change your life.)

The purpose of this book is nothing less than to provide you with the tools to return to a state of freedom. To restore your body and confidence to live the life you once lived before your back troubles robbed you of it. Rest assured that the tools in this book are rooted in science. They are the result of information drawn from brilliant researchers and clinicians, distilled into accessible concepts that are simple and easy to follow. I personally incorporate the lessons highlighted in this book into my daily life, and I teach them to all my clients. Whether they are professional athletes or everyday working folks, the results are outstanding. Thanks to Jeremy and Chris, you, too, now have a complete guide to spine health — and a program that will change your life.

This book has it right. It is a must-read for anyone who wishes to reverse or prevent serious back pain. Read it closely. It contains the core concepts and corrective measures that are essential to creating a more resilient spine. Work hard on the exercises and pay special attention to the behavioral habits that Jeremy emphasizes. There is every reason to hope that you will experience blessed, permanent relief. The tools are here. Use them and move on to a great, pain-free life.

BILL FABROCINI, PT, CSCS

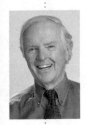

## CHAPTER ONE

# The Promise

### From Chris

Back pain is the monster in most of our lives. The ogre under the bed. The ogre that lands *you* in bed all too often. Or on the floor . . . flopping around in pain. Like a sunfish on a hot cement dock.

Most Americans know that pain well. Know the agony, the sudden sickening return after it's been gone for a while. The canceling of plans, the loss of a job. Everything. They cannot *live* with it—not really live—and they would do anything for relief. But there is no relief. They've tried everything, and nothing works. Nothing meaningful, anyway. Back pain sufferers spend an average of $2,500 a year for palliative "fixes," but they get precious little in return. They'd spend more—they'd spend *anything*—if the fixes really worked. But most don't. Or not very well. Or not for long. People structure their lives around the pain as best they can, but that doesn't work either, because you never know when it's going to hit.

And when it comes, it's not like a sore shoulder or a bum leg; you can't use the other arm instead. You can't limp along with a cane, relying on the good leg. When your back is the problem, everything goes, and you're *cooked. When your back hurts, your life hurts. And you can't do a damned thing.*

## THE PROMISE

That is about to end. You are going to have trouble believing that sentence, but it's *true.* That pain is about to go away or be sharply reduced. And the change is going to be permanent. For about 80 percent of you, anyway. That's an astonishing promise, and it's absolutely true. We know of nothing else in the field that comes close.

*"Success" means either the permanent elimination of pain (the result for most of you) or a reduction of its severity from the 7–10 level—on a scale of 1–10* (that's *agony)—to the 1–3 level* (that's a nuisance). Blessed, blessed relief, either way. As I say, it is only going to work for about 80 percent of you, but that's a near-miracle. And Jeremy has solid suggestions for the rest of you, too. (See Chapter 4 to learn if you're in the 20 percent and find out what to do.) *But remember the main point: For 80 percent of you, the pain stops here.*

We hope that the "you" in that sentence is an enormous number of people. Jeremy is a modest man but he *knows* what he can do—what he has done—and he is ambitious about taking his protocol to a much broader audience. Indeed, he wants to start a revolution in back pain care in America, starting with you, and he wants it to be universal and cheap. He thinks—he and I think—that it can be done in a book. That sounds wild—that this horrendous problem can be fixed with such a modest tool. But it's not. Because back pain is all about *behavior,* and you can deal with *behavior* in a book. As you will learn in a moment, the vast majority of you created your back pain *with* your own, long-term *behavior.* And only *you* can fix it, with profound changes in that *behavior*. It is a matter of showing you what you did before that made a mess of your back, and teaching you what you have to do now. And then you doing it. Jeremy explains, and he shows you how. You do the work. You *will* succeed. A surprise, perhaps one you will have trouble getting your head around at first. But it's true: You *will* succeed.

So how bad is the problem? Pretty bad, as most of you know. Four out of five of us have back pain so bad we seek help from health care professionals. The nation as a whole spends $100 billion on the problem. It does more to disrupt business than anything else. And, of course, it raises hell with millions of lives. For some, it is a recurring nuisance, something that takes the joy out of the day, the week, the month. For more of us, it is an intermittent horror, with the pain at the agony level and we just can't move. Your wife calls your host for dinner: "Bill is flat on his back on the floor. We may have to go to the hospital. Sorry." You can't go out to dinner; you can't perform your duties. Hell, you can't get off the floor! It ruins careers, messes up companies, trashes marriages, and raises holy hell with just about everything else. For most, it comes and goes, but when it comes . . . *it's just god-awful*. Oh *lord!* What do you do?

Not much, until now. There's conventional medicine—which is such a blessing in so many areas of our lives—but it is apt not to be great for back pain. For extreme cases (the 20 percent we mentioned), there is surgery, and for them it may be the only option; Jeremy will alert those who should be thinking about it. But surgery—tremendously important and successful for some—is not the answer for most of you. It is well known, for example, that at least one popular operation—spinal fusion— is one of the most overprescribed operations in the country. It is a serious operation (it costs about $100,000), it is often unnecessary, and it often doesn't work. Not for long, anyway, and sometimes not at all. That is scary. Jeremy, and the best surgeons, all say that surgery should be a last resort. There are other "medical" steps, like cortisone or other shots, but, once again, relief is temporary, there can be serious side effects, and there are limits to how often you can go there. The basic problem with traditional medicine and back pain is that they are not a very good fit. Western medicine is not heavily focused on behavioral problems and behavioral change; it simply did not grow up that way. And back pain is primarily a behavioral problem. Which means that, ultimately, only you can fix it.

Don't worry if this concept doesn't quite sink in at the first reading. It's what the whole book is about. We'll get there. Together.

### A Younger Next Year Book

I say "we'll get there together," and that's an important part of the book and the cure. This is "a Younger Next Year" book. That means several things, as some of you know. First, it means there is a presentation by *two writers*, a deadly serious professional scientist (that's Jeremy for this book . . . it was Harry Lodge in the first Younger Next Year books) and a layman (me). As I used to say of Harry and as I now say of Jeremy: "He's young and smart, and I'm old and funny." The pairing is supposed to make the book easier to follow (and maybe just a teeny bit fun to read) without losing a whisper of scientific integrity. The scientist is in charge throughout, but reading the book should not make your teeth hurt. Not hurt badly, anyway.

It also means that the core idea is that *behavioral change* can have a profound effect on your wellness and quality of life. Far more of an effect, in important areas, than the best conventional medicine. The "modest" boast in the original *Younger Next Year* book was that behavioral change could put off *70 percent of aging* until close to the end of life, and *eliminate 50 percent of the most serious diseases completely*. Which was absolutely true; no one has ever disagreed. Over 2 million people bought *Younger Next Year* (in twenty-three languages) and made it a cult book for those over forty, many thousands of whom profoundly changed their lives. A huge number of people have come up to me and Harry over the years to say, "Hey, man, thanks for writing that book; it changed my life." Nice.

The *Younger Next Year Back Book* is a little more specific: *Behavioral change*—spelled out by Jeremy—*can end or radically reduce back pain*. But the consequences for back pain sufferers are every bit as important. I was with Jeremy recently when a guy in his fifties said to me that he'd come to Jeremy the previous summer, after a lifetime of serious back pain: "I could not bend over to lace my own shoes. I'd been in agony for decades. And Jeremy simply fixed it. Jeremy gave me my life back." Jeremy has a thousand stories like that. More than a thousand. We hope to have a million before we're done.

Finally, it means that the book has a certain integrity. Harry and I went to great lengths to make *Younger Next Year* solid—conservative, if anything. To the best of our knowledge, there was not a single exaggeration, and certainly not a single misstatement. Jeremy and I have done the same here. Dealing with back pain is an evolving field, and some things we say may turn out to be wrong as people learn more. But not the basic lines and not the major claims. The book is as solid as we can make it, and it will stand up. As *Younger Next Year* has done, strikingly.

Jeremy came to me with the idea for doing this book together because he thought *YNY* and his story had "the same genes." Which was quite right. Beyond that, Jeremy is a "good guy"; he wants to do good in this world, and the fact that back pain makes such a mess of so many lives—unnecessarily in his view—makes him crazy. He knew how successful the Younger Next Year books had been, he knew me, and he thought that maybe the two of us could pair up and *get the word out . . . change the world of back pain.*

So that's our modest goal here—first Jeremy's and now mine: We just want to, you know, change the world. And eliminate back pain for millions. Hey, couldn't hurt. Along the way we hope to make a couple of billion dollars ourselves but Jeremy's great motivation is to change the world of back pain. Pretty good guy, Jeremy.

Now, let's have a quiet word about some things this book won't do. It won't do any good if you just stick it under your pillow, for example. You have to read it. Closely. We'll make that as easy as we can but it ain't always going to be a walk on the beach. *Then*, by heaven, you have to go to work *yourself* on the cure. You have to do the initial fixes yourself. And then you have to adopt Jeremy's carefully tailored exercise regimen to make the cure permanent, and that's not always easy. Well, it's easy if you know how, and we work like crazy to show you how in the book (and in videos we'll refer to in a minute).

Finally, you have to know—as I said before—that the book may not work for some of you. You're too far gone. Awfully damn sorry about that but about 20 percent of you—Jeremy estimates, conservatively—are going to have progressed to a stage where you are probably going to need traditional medical help, possibly including surgery. He'll tell you how to know if that means you. And a few more of you—with back pain that is rooted primarily in muscle "trigger points" (there's a terrific chapter on that)—may need to turn to a chiropractor or physical therapist, at least briefly, to show you how to find and release muscle spasms. Then you come back to the book to lock in the change and make it permanent. But the basic claim—that some 80 percent of you can get complete or significant pain relief permanently—is solid.

I asked Jeremy, early on, if he could back up that number by going through his records. He said he could not. (Oh, lord!) *But*, he said, he could remember every single one of the handful of patients he thought he could help who in fact he could not (excluding the ones he sent on for conventional medical help). He could count them on his fingers. I thought that was good enough. So, that 80 percent claim is not just solid, it is conservative.

## Basic Insight: You Got Yourself into This Mess, and Only You Can Get Yourself Out

Jeremy's success has been based on two great insights. The first was to realize (along with a handful of others, including Bill Fabrocini, who wrote the Introduction) that *your own long-term behavior* (how you carry yourself, your posture, and certain repetitive movements) is almost always the *cause* of your back pain. Sometimes it's trauma or a weird event but not often. And only *changing behavior* is going to effect a *permanent cure*. In other words, it's going to be up to you in the end. Jeremy will point the way and tell you exactly what to do: first to effect the cure and then to do maintenance. But you do the hard work. And—as in the other Younger Next Year books—exercise is going to be at the heart of it. Steady, whole-body exercise for the rest of your life. If you're new to all this, that may sound alarming—steady exercise forever—but it's not. In this, as in other things, exercise is going to turn out to be the key to the good life.

The second great insight was to realize that, while back pain *seems* local and specific, it is almost always a *whole-body* or at least *whole-core* problem in the end (we'll tell you all about the core in a bit). And *a whole-body approach* is indispensable to its cure. Drawing on those two insights, on his review of the available science, and on his own vast, clinical experience (he has been doing nothing but treating back pain his whole adult life), Jeremy has developed a technique that has had unprecedented success.

You are probably a bit of a student of back pain yourself if you've had it for a while, but you are about to learn some new things. You will learn, for example, that back pain is not a "disease," as some doctors say. Nor, in most cases, is it the result of an accident or trauma. Or bad genes or bad luck. Or (mostly) psychological issues. Sometimes, but mostly not. And it is not from rolling over "funny" in the night or picking up something heavy, carelessly. Or making love in some goofy and disgusting way. It's not the malfunction of a particular disc or vertebra or a spasm in a particular muscle, although it almost always "reads" that way. A particular disc, spasm, or whatnot is the *immediate* source of the pain. But that's not what it's all about. Almost all back pain is a "whole-body" problem, certainly a "whole-spine and core" problem, caused by the way we live and move, over time. Caused by our rotten posture, by sitting curled over a computer eight hours a day for *years and years*, by our idleness, by the shameful weakness of our core. And—a close corollary of the foregoing—by the foolish ways we *move*, day in and day out. Fix those big problems *carefully* and the little problems, which actually cause the specific pain, go away.

What we are going to do first, after giving you a background tour of your spine and its discontents, is teach you to find and maintain a neutral spine (the position that allows your spine to do its job with the least amount of stress and load–and the least damage) all the time. Don't worry if that term doesn't mean anything to you now; it will mean a lot by the time we're done. It is the first and last key to your recovery. Then we're going to show you how to use the core to *support* the neutral spine. Next, we're going to teach you exercises to increase the strength and endurance of the core so it can do its primary job, which turns out to be supporting the neutral spine in the long term and keeping it *stable*. Finally, we're going to teach you to avoid triggering behaviors (like playing golf a certain way or bending over your computer for twenty years). Teach you *how to move correctly*, so that you maintain a neutral and stable spine all the time, even when doing the complex lifting and rotating motions that are part of daily life and exercise. We're going to teach you how to *behave*, frankly. And back pain will significantly *go away*. Easy-peasy.

You will want to know that Jeremy understands the specific problems—the disc bulges, the "pinched" nerves, the muscle spasms, and all that—as well as anyone in the professions, and we'll talk a good deal about those along the way. But his over-arching insight is that it is a mistake to focus on those. Rather, he wants us to make fundamental (but manageable) behavioral changes that affect our entire core, our entire body. Then the specific problems that are making us crazy go away. Indeed, fundamental behavioral change is the *only* way to effect permanent change. Otherwise, local "fixes"—like spinal fusions, laminectomies, discectomies . . . all the stuff you've heard about from your medical doctor—will usually offer only temporary relief. Blessed relief but temporary. The overall problem persists. And it will turn up in the abutting vertebrae or at another place down the kinetic chain (the complex chain of joints, discs, and connective tissue in and around the spine). Conventional medicine performs wonders. Obviously. And it has a huge role in acute situations. But it generally cannot achieve lifelong *cures* for chronic back pain. Only *you* can do that, and only with behavioral change and a certain exercise regimen. Jeremy can show you how.

Jeremy wants me to stress that we are most assuredly not putting down modern medicine. He comes from a long line of doctors, and he has the liveliest sense that modern medicine is miraculous. But there are areas where medicine is limited to fixing *but not curing* problems, areas where behavioral change matters much more. Heart disease is one of them, interestingly enough. And back pain is another.

A closing word: Trees are bent by prevailing winds. Bodies are bent by prevailing postures and movements. Trees can live in their contorted condition. Bodies cannot. Our bodies are meant to stand erect on the earth. When they do not, they cry out to us. They cry out in pain.

## A NOTE ABOUT VIDEOS

If you are a visual learner, you may want to take a look at Jeremy's program of streamed videos (BackForever.com) on aspects of back pain. See the appendix for information. BackForever.com is *by no means a substitute* for the book, but it offers a different angle on the subject and some additional information that may be helpful.

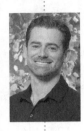

## CHAPTER TWO

# Jeremy's Story

**From Jeremy**

got into the business of healing back pain because I had serious back pain myself, as a young man, caused by a series of athletic injuries. I got into chiropractic and related whole-body disciplines because nothing else worked for me. I went on to develop my own, very different variations on familiar chiropractic practices over time. I do not "pop" backs or any of that, but I draw heavily on the basic elements of the discipline, as well as my reading of the scientific literature generally and my own considerable experience as a practitioner.

I grew up in a traditional medical household, and fully expected to go to medical school and then into practice. My grandfather was a medical doctor, my father is a medical doctor, my mom is a nurse, my aunt is a nurse, my uncle was a pharmaceutical salesman. I was as deeply immersed in traditional Western medicine as one could possibly be, and I had—and still have—tremendous respect for it. When I was little, I was used to having people come up to me and tell me how much my grandfather had done to save this or that child from some grim fate. He was one of those doctors that they don't really make anymore. He performed surgeries, delivered babies, made house calls, and was a master diagnostician. And he was also a terrific guy whom I admired a lot. Later I heard the same things about my parents from their patients.

So I grew up believing there wasn't much that modern medicine could not fix, and I couldn't wait to become a part of it. I emphasize all this because, eventually, I am going to sound a bit reserved about traditional Western medicine and back pain, and I don't want you to be confused: I revere traditional medicine and understand it better than most. It's just that it generally isn't great at curing back pain. And back pain is what I had as a young man . . . a lot of it. And it has been my life ever since.

## My Personal Pain: Part One

When I was a teenager, I thought I was going to be a professional skateboarder. If you are over fifty, do not snap the book closed at this point; skateboarding is a terrific sport. But it is a slightly dangerous sport and I took many, many falls, some of them pretty bad. I did not become a professional skateboarder; I might have been good enough, but long before that could happen I became a very young man with extremely serious back pain. When that happened, I went the traditional medical route. I went to regular doctors (good ones, as you'd expect) and was poked and prodded; I had ultrasounds and MRIs and blood tests and you-name-it. They talked about an extraordinary range of possible causes, including "slipped discs," "ruptured discs," "pinched nerves," maybe cancer. Wow! But they could not fix my pain. I was somewhat medically astute, even as a kid, and I became increasingly convinced that a lot of these well-meaning, well-trained doctors didn't really know an awful lot about my back pain. Sounds harsh, but it has turned out to be true of quite a few conventional doctors.

In near desperation, I turned to less traditional medicine—to chiropractors. And darned if I didn't find at least some symptomatic relief. That was huge, and it opened my head to the possibility of going in that direction. I should mention that those particular chiropractors weren't perfect, either. They didn't begin to teach me how to make fundamental changes. They didn't talk about changing my own behaviors or suggest how to take control of my own health or do any of the things that are at the heart of my practice today. But they did show me that the pain could be affected with simple muscle and joint work, and I was deeply impressed by that. Chiropractic treatment has its place in back care and offers many benefits when done properly. Skilled chiropractors use manual (with their hands) therapy to restore normal joint movement and muscle function through chiropractic adjustments and other techniques such as stretching and joint mobilization. This therapy can be invaluable, especially in the short term. But even today many chiropractors do not teach their patients how to make the necessary behavioral changes to permanently relieve back pain.

I decided to train in chiropractic, because I wanted to dig deeper into what I already recognized as the real causes—and perhaps the real treatment—of serious back pain: behavior and behavioral change. That drove my very medical family crazy, as you can imagine, but in retrospect it was exactly the right decision.

My education was a long and complex process. I took guidance from a range of experts in the chiropractic and other fields. But I eventually developed my own analyses and my own approach to permanently ending back pain in my patients.

Traditional medicine takes a basically *deconstructivist* approach: It generally takes complex problems apart, analyzes the pieces with exquisite care, then identifies and cures the particular problem. That deconstructivist approach works miraculously for many, many medical problems, but not for back pain. For back pain you want an *integrationist* approach. You want whole-body solutions.

## My Personal Pain: Part Two

I had a second round of back pain, long after I should have known better, and I want to tell you that embarrassing story for several reasons. First, because the pain was so dreadful, and I want you to know just how deeply I understand and empathize with significant pain. Second, I want to stress just how vulnerable *all* of us are to default behaviors that can raise holy hell with our backs, including people like me, who surely should have known better. And third, I want to show how quickly and effectively you can deal with even the gravest back pain, once you know what you're doing.

The time is seven years ago. I was working part of the time on a very promising medical start-up venture. For six months, I was absolutely obsessed with it. I worked regular ten- and twelve-hour days with few breaks for leisure or exercise. Most of the time, I was bent over my computer. I worked like an absolute lunatic and did not think twice about my back. Pathetic.

One morning, after a particularly grueling stretch of days and nights, I woke up at six and started to sit up to go to the john. I was smacked by the most ferocious pain I've ever had in my life, even worse than anything from my skateboarding days. I was knocked flat on my back and could not budge. Even when I was lying absolutely still, the pain continued, unabated, at a fierce level. If I tried to move, it was much, much worse. I lived alone back then, and all I could do was lie there and wonder, in near panic: What in the world is going on? Just how bad is this? Am I going to die, for heaven's sake? Not only was I in terrible pain; I was seriously scared.

I remembered how "normal" back pain felt, a bad spasm or whatever. But this seemed to be way beyond that. So what was it? A ruptured disc would be the good news. At the other end of the spectrum, perhaps it was some weird cancer, somewhere in my spine.

That was ridiculous, but truly severe pain leads to some wild and unpredictable thoughts. I was sweating and breathing hard and was on the edge of panic. And that went on for what seemed like forever. At last my long scientific training and experience took over. The first step was to ask myself the questions I ask all my patients: How did this happen? What "behavior" might have caused this? It's interesting just how often the sufferer knows intuitively what he or she had done (at least the triggering event) and I was no different. It did not take long to conclude that it was probably those months of nonstop work, bent over a computer. Of course! For someone with my history, that was nuts. And step one was to *stop doing what had caused the pain in the first place.* (If I ever managed to sit or stand again.) The problem right now was to ease the pain and move. With more than a little agony, I rolled onto my side to see if I could stand. I couldn't. The pain ratcheted up to new levels and slapped me flat on my back again. It felt as if someone were stabbing me in my kidneys and dragging the knife down into my buttocks. It literally took my breath away.

Then it was back to basics: I did what I always do in those relatively rare cases when I'm there during a patient's attack. I told myself to tense my abdominal muscles a little and slowly pick up my left foot. I am lying flat in bed and picking up one foot, just a little bit. That simple first step, which I have counseled so many times, was bearable. It almost always is. I set that foot down and picked up the right foot, continuing to tense my abdominal muscles. That also was doable. Good. Then on to the next phase: I walked carefully, very gently, in place—lying on my back and not lifting my feet very far—for perhaps five minutes. The pain slowly lessened. I stopped, and did it again several times. I was "walking off" the pain. *And* I was easing what almost certainly was a particularly bad muscle spasm, somewhere near my lumbar spine.

Eventually, I felt ready to stand. I lightly tensed the muscles in my abdomen to support my spine and keep it still and rolled onto my side. As you will soon learn, this tensing of those muscles is called locking down or engaging your core. This time I could do it. I was careful to keep my lower back *still* and my abdomen braced throughout the movement. It was not pain-free, but I made it to my knees, then my feet. I was mighty careful to keep my lumbar spine still and my core engaged throughout, because I knew that, in the wake of an attack like this, the spasm and the pain were just waiting to come roaring back. Then I tried walking erect. And, yes, I could walk. I walked back and forth across the room carefully, keeping my core tight. I did that for quite a while and the spasm and pain calmed down.

For the rest of that day, I was very careful about how I moved, and my back continued to get better. I knew from experience that those first steps would work because I had taught them to so many others. For the rest of the day, I took it easy and did no more than a little easy walking. By tomorrow, I assured myself, my back will slowly loosen up. It will take a week to return to normal, because the spasm was so strong. But in a week, I will be there. Then I will resume my regular exercise regimen, and stick to it religiously. I will not sit at the computer for more than thirty minutes at a time without taking a break and walking around. And so on and so forth. In fact, I did all that. In a week, I was moving and living normally. I did not let the intensity of my work interfere with my exercise regimen ever again. And the pain never returned.

With my horror story behind us, I want to visit four other sufferers. But first, let Chris take you on a stroll down your own spine, and tell you about how your spine works and how it can go wrong.

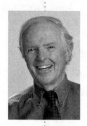

## CHAPTER THREE

# A Walk Down Your Spine

**From Chris**

Congratulations, you're a vertebrate. You, sir . . . you, madam . . . have a backbone. Nice going.

I know there are times when you're writhing on the floor in agony—that sunfish-on-the-hot-dock thing—because the back pain's so awful. That's when having a backbone doesn't seem so great. But it really is. The alternative is being a jellyfish or an amoeba, little guys like that. No back pain but no fun, either. The backbone is one of the great keys to having fun, having a life. Unless, of course, it gets messed up. Then it's the great key to agony.

The object of this ambitious little book is to give you the key to eliminating or drastically reducing back pain, now and forever. And sharply increasing the fun. If Jeremy knows what he's talking about (and he does), you will do those things through new knowledge and behavioral change. First, by understanding what's been going on back there, all this time. And then by changing how you carry yourself, how you move, and how you exercise. Jeremy throws new light on all this and makes it easy. Sort of easy. Easier than that sunfish-on-the-dock business anyway. That's pretty bad.

Okay, step one toward "knowing what's been going on back there" is a little "walk down your back" to show you how the sucker works. Why, you may ask, is a Wall Street lawyer writing this chapter? Two reasons: First, it shows that *anyone* can understand it. Second, this stuff can be a teeny bit dull, and the theory is that I can help with that. Not much, but some.

Start with the basics. The development of the vertebrate spine, which we share with all living creatures of any size, was perhaps the second biggest breakthrough in all evolution (after the brain). It lets us do *everything*: stand, run, make love, move in all the amazing ways we move. It is a truly astonishing and wonderful thing. It *does* get screwed up once in a while. And it's extraordinarily complicated. But here's the deal: Solving the horror of back pain is nowhere near as complicated as you might logically assume, given how complex your back is. That's the magic of Jeremy's way and of this little book: While the spine and its contributing parts are exquisitely complex (as you're about to read), solving back pain is surprisingly simple. The problems vary tremendously from person to person and from back to back. But the solutions to most of the problems are the same. And they are pretty simple. That may be hard to believe, but it's true. That phenomenon is at the heart of his 80 percent cure rate.

Let's begin by getting you oriented. It's tempting to talk "cure" from the beginning, and I guess we could. But it's our sense that you will get more out of this if you have a pretty good understanding of what your back is like and how it works. Then Jeremy gets down to making yours work right.

Here is an important conceptual issue, one of the most important in the book. Laypeople like you and me tend to think of the back as the spine—the pile of bones and discs that we see in all the charts. And in the grim skeleton that hangs in the doctor's office. That's not totally dumb, but it's misleading. Jeremy sees (and heals) your back quite differently, and you will, too, when we're done. He sees it as a thoroughly integrated "whole," because it works as a whole and gets messed up as a whole. In the end, it is not the individual pieces that get fouled up, as we tend to assume; it's the "system." And when he says "the whole," he means *the works*. He sees your back as pretty much everything between your head and your legs, on the front, sides, and back of your body: bones, discs, nerves, muscles, tendons and ligaments, circulation—the whole shebang.

Does that make sense? Well, yeah, it does. Because in fact all those elements really do work together all the time, and if you focus on the parts rather than *the functioning whole*, you're going to get things wrong. As Jeremy said: Regular Western medicine is much given to focusing on the parts, not the whole— the "deconstructionist" approach. That's its great gift, the ability to home in on tiny details. But regular Western medicine is not so hot at fixing back pain, because, with back pain, the devil is not in the details. As we were careful to say at the outset, we're not here to pick fights with regular Western medicine, which is breathtakingly good at all kinds of things, sometimes including back pain. But not always. Because a real cure for back pain is almost always a matter of *profound, whole-body, behavioral change*, and modern medicine is not in the business of behavioral change. It should be but it isn't, although changes are afoot.

## The Spinal Cord

Let's start with the innermost tissues—the spinal cord, which comes down *inside* the pile of bones, the vertebrae—and work our way out to the skin. The spinal cord is the critical bundle of nerves that runs from the brain, down the middle of the spine, and out to the muscles and everywhere else. It has the consistency of an unripe banana and, if it is bruised, to say nothing of cut, it *never* recovers; you're in that wheelchair or whatever for the rest of your life. If a nerve's axon is severed, the nerve will not heal or grow back. This is unlike damaged muscles, skin, and bone. My beloved wife, Hilary, broke her neck badly (at C5–6, if you know about such things), soon after we were married, so we learned this terrifying message in depth. Turns out, she was one in a thousand (literally) to walk, after an injury like hers (her X-rays are in medical texts). We were astonishingly lucky and had amazing care. But the lesson stands: The spinal column is vulnerable and the body will go to weird lengths to protect it. Some of those lengths cause back pain.

The spinal cord is hugely important. It is the information highway that sends messages to, and receives messages from, the muscles and everything else. In the end, your body is a giant signaling system, with billions and billions of signals running up and down your spine and then all over the place to tell you to move, feel, breathe, digest, and do pretty much everything we do. Most of those signals start out in your brain and run down your spinal cord. That cord, as I say, is tucked away for safety in the middle of the spinal column, the chain of (hollow) bones or vertebrae running down your back. The nerves jump off at various stages, along your spine. Those little jumping-off places (holes in the spine, or "foramina") are rich with possibilities of things going wrong as your back gets bent out of shape (by the silly way you walk and carry yourself) and causing you pain. A *ton* of it. The picture on page 26 (showing the major nerves coming out of the spine) gives you a broad idea.

*Here is some good news: This chapter looks hard, but it is not. It is merely designed to give you an overall background on the subject, and you don't have to remember a damned thing. That's what makes it easy.* All you and I need to know about nerves and foramina and all that, for example, is that there are a lot of nerves and groups of nerves coming off the spinal column at various points and that they are vulnerable at those points. The spine, with its various exits at different levels, is an intricate, exquisitely "machined" system with little margin for error. So your "back" has to be working smoothly if this nervous system is to work right. If it doesn't work right, it hurts. Like crazy.

**The Nervous System**

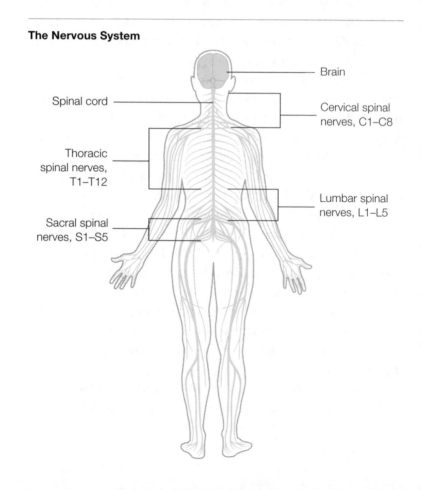

Spinal cord

Thoracic
spinal nerves,
T1–T12

Sacral spinal
nerves, S1–S5

Brain

Cervical spinal
nerves, C1–C8

Lumbar spinal
nerves, L1–L5

If it gets compressed or twisted in some goofy way over time, because, say, the way you carry yourself is dumb, it's gonna hurt. *That is all you really need to know. Relax.*

In addition to the thick rope of nerves that constitutes the spinal cord, there are zillions of nerves that service the spine itself. Call them "local" nerves. And guess what? They can hurt, too, if you mess with them. The picture on the opposite page shows the spinal cord and the nerves branching out from it and going all over.

## The Spine

Okay, that's the child's version of the spinal cord or superhighway of nerves. Now we get to talk about the spine—the bones and discs—which is actually the foundation upon which your body is built. The keel of your boat, or however you want to think of it. And its extraordinary gift is that, unlike the keel of your boat or the foundation of your house, it is *flexible*. Actually, it is better than that: It is rigid, much of the time. Which allows you to sit and stand upright and be stable, even under great pressure, while the hips and shoulders allow you to move and perform tasks. But it can also bend, forward and back and from side to side, when you need it to do that. And even twist a little. Amazing. It is "articulated" like a linked chain. Which is to say, it is made up of a bunch of pieces and they let you flex. The individual pieces are the bones, called vertebrae—some thirty-three of them—stacked on top of each other with semisoft shock absorbers or "discs" in between them. The spine is divided into sections based on the curvature of the spine in each section. The four sections are the cervical spine (neck), thoracic spine (upper and mid back), lumbar spine (lower back), and sacrum and coccyx (tailbone). Different nerves stem out of the spine at different places and go on to regulate specific parts of your body. This may interest me more than most, but that's why, if you break your back and damage your spine up high, almost all the nerves are affected and almost nothing "works"—you are apt to be a quadriplegic. If the damage happens lower down, your upper body works okay, but you can't walk. If it happens really high on your neck, you can't breathe; you're on a respirator.

All the bones in the spine are movable and have discs in between them except the sacrum and coccyx, which are fused or sealed together (no discs for them, of course). The discs, which we'll come to in a moment, are, according to Jeremy, "made up of a fibrous outer layer, which resists fraying or breaking under normal conditions, and an inner liquid core called the nucleus pulposus, which gives the discs the ability to distribute loads evenly throughout the discs and resist compressive forces." I like to think of them as very tough jelly doughnuts: They are tough on the outside and have goo or jelly on the inside, so they can give with pressure and rebound. They can be compressed, angled, and so on, but not endlessly. We'll come back to that in a moment. Abused or bulging discs can hurt like crazy. Ruptured discs are much worse.

*Here is an important home truth.* The whole spine is articulated but not to the same degree. Most urgently, your lower or lumbar spine—the area that most often gets messed up—isn't meant to handle loads in flexed or rotated positions. Do those words make any sense to you? What they mean, in the end, is *Don't bend, lift, and twist with your lower back.* There. That is one of the most important lessons in the book. Your lumbar spine is designed to hold you up, almost as if it were fused. We need to have some movement in there, but not much, and certainly not with loads, especially repetitive loads. The little muscles around it are meant to keep it stable, not to lift things, and so on.

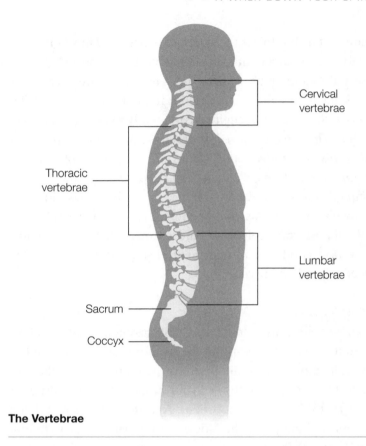

Cervical
vertebrae

Thoracic
vertebrae

Lumbar
vertebrae

Sacrum

Coccyx

**The Vertebrae**

Put it this way, as if it came from the Decalogue: *Thou shalt not rotate with thy lower back.* Rotate with your hips, not your lower back. How do you rotate with your hips instead of your lower back? Easy. We will show you.

**THE HOLY GRAIL**
Again, we're getting ahead of ourselves, but the simple picture above shows the neutral spine position. That's the Holy Grail in this book—maintaining a neutral spine. This is the way you want to carry yourself, almost all the time. Jeremy will talk about it in

greater detail, but this is the safest, strongest, and most effective way to carry yourself and support loads. It may be a slight surprise, but "standing up straight" does not mean your neutral or ideal spine is straight: it is a series of natural curves. Why? Who knows. Ask a structural engineer, preferably a suspension bridge builder. *What I have learned from Jeremy (and Bill, before him) is that this is the ideal, and it is worth going to a tremendous amount of trouble to get into the habit of carrying yourself in this position.* I now think about it all the time—sitting, walking, riding my bike, in spin class—*all* the time. I can *feel* it, when I am in the right posture; it feels good. And, it turns out, that's a blessing. If you take good care of your neutral spine, it will go very far indeed toward taking care of you.

## IT'S HOLLOW!

I confess, with only a touch of embarrassment, that I had no idea until we started working on this book that each vertebra was really a two-part bone. There is the more or less solid and weight-bearing portion toward your front, called "the vertebral body" (with the discs in between). And then there's this flying buttress–looking piece that sticks off the back (the "vertebral arch"). And there is a very important space between the two sections. The "hollow" down the middle of your spine is really a space between these two segments of the vertebra. The vertebra is one solid piece of bone but with two very distinct segments and a hole down the middle where the spinal cord goes.

Do you see the spiny-looking pieces in the next picture, on page 32, sticking off the vertebrae? Those are pieces of the vertebral arch. They are called "the spinous processes" (no one cares), and they are basically anchor points. That's where ligaments can attach muscles to the vertebrae. If you're a sailor, think of cleats on the deck, for ropes. When you reach back and feel the spiny part of your back, you're feeling the "spinous processes" or the cleats. By the way, the ligaments or sinews are the lines (think "stays" on a sailboat) that hold your spine erect. Without stays, the mast on a sailboat would flop around and break in no time; with stays, the mast on a well-designed sailboat is remarkably stable. Flexible, like your spine, but stable and strong, too.

Okeydoke, on to the discs. This is familiar territory to most of us. You hear about discs all the time. "Bulging discs," "pinched discs," "slipped discs," "ruptured discs" and so on. They are basically washers to keep the weight-bearing parts of the vertebrae from rubbing on one another and to put some "give" into your back. You cannot have an articulated stack of bones without a wonderfully effective stack of washers to keep 'em apart, and you do. Think of them as very tough jelly doughnuts, as I mentioned before. There is a tough, fibrous layer on the outside and a gooey or liquid core on the inside. They act as shock absorbers and have a lot to do with letting you bend. Dysfunctional discs can be a major source of problems and pain.

## A YOUNG PERSON'S PROBLEMS

This is interesting. Bulging and actually ruptured discs are mostly a young person's problem, people in their thirties (and you kids are welcome to them; they *really* hurt). Older people have horrendous problems, too; after all, some 35 percent of people from ages forty-five to sixty-five have serious back pain. But usually not this particular horror. Which also means that more younger people are going to get bundled off to the surgeon, if the problem is grim enough. Older people have disc problems, too, but nowhere near as often.

Take a long look at the pictures on the next pages. They show you how the spinal cord, spine, and discs work together. First is a side view depicting how the brain, spinal cord, and spine are positioned in the body. Second is a close-up of a segment made up of two vertebrae with their disc (in gray) in between and the spinal cord and nerve roots visible. Notice how the rear parts of the adjoining vertebrae form a canal through which the spinal cord runs from top to bottom. Also notice how the two adjoining vertebrae form holes, or "foramina," on the sides where the nerve roots come out of the spine. Those holes are super-important: The holes can become smaller from disc degeneration or movement of the vertebrae on top of each other. And the nerve that comes out of the hole is pressured, and it hurts like blazes. Not to get too scary, but when things really go to hell and you actually *rupture* or split the disc open with your ridiculous posture or whatnot, the pain really goes over the top. (Good news: You hear about ruptured discs all the time, but they are comparatively rare.) Bones wear on bones, discs hurt like crazy, and the stuff in the middle squirts all over the place. Which is bad because it

**The Spinal Column**

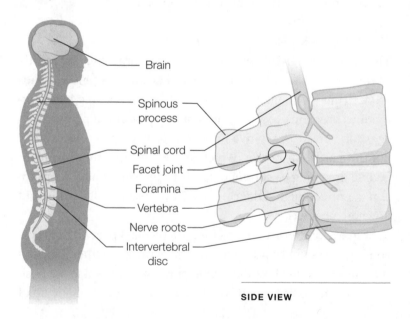

Brain

Spinous process

Spinal cord

Facet joint

Foramina

Vertebra

Nerve roots

Intervertebral disc

**SIDE VIEW**

causes severe *chemical* pain in the nerves. Not so good. When we say that there are times when traditional medicine (surgery) has a critical role, this is one of them.

Note the bits of bone to the left in the close-up side view vertebral segment. These are "the facet joints." The point of this picture is to show how they are right next to the spinal cord and near one of the nerve exit spots. They are well placed, in other words, to raise hell if things go wrong with them. I forgot to mention this: The surfaces of the facet joints are covered in cartilage, which allows smooth movement in a healthy spine. So what? The point is that this cartilage can be abraded or torn by dumb moves, too, and that hurts as well.

Here are two more views, below. Note the sort of circular thing with the lighter insides. That's a cross section of a disc, seen from the top.

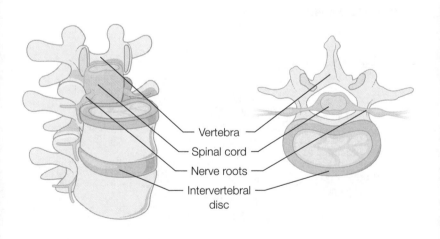

Vertebra
Spinal cord
Nerve roots
Intervertebral disc

**THREE-QUARTER VIEW**          **TOP VIEW**

## Ligaments and Tendons

All right, that's the spinal cord and the spinal column. But they would not stand alone without a ton of support. Think of the spinal column as a slender reed. If you press down on it at all from above (or the sides), it will bend crazily. Indeed, it cannot sustain any weight at all to speak of. But now, add a bunch of support lines from the pole to a solid support, and it's a different story. Our backbone has a lot of very sturdy support lines called ligaments and tendons (ligaments connect bone to bone; tendons connect bone to muscle.) There are an awful lot of ligaments connected to the spine. The following picture gives you the idea.

Here's another thing you need to know: Ligaments can become deformed or *sprained* because of bad posture, a persistent pattern of bad movements, or an injury. When that happens to a ligament, the joints those ligaments were supporting "get loose" and can slip around. That is really bad. Here is a language

**Spinal Ligaments**

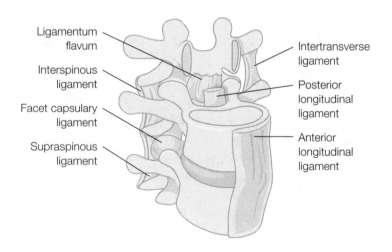

Ligamentum flavum

Interspinous ligament

Facet capsulary ligament

Supraspinous ligament

Intertransverse ligament

Posterior longitudinal ligament

Anterior longitudinal ligament

alert: A "sprain" is an unhealthy stretch or tear of a ligament, and a "strain" is an unhealthy stretch or tear in a tendon or muscle. Look at the picture on the opposite page: there are a ton of ligaments here, all waiting to go haywire if you are foolish or unlucky.

All right, that's it for bones, discs, and ligaments. *What was the point?* Good question. The whole point of that part of the walk down the spine was to give you a detailed sense of just how complicated the spine and all its elements really are and how easily—and variously—they can go wrong. And hurt. But let me repeat myself on this key point: The essence of Jeremy's remarkable technique is that it does *not* focus on the details of what has gone wrong. It focuses on the *whole*. Your very complicated back is an integrated whole. Integrated with your muscles, too, which we haven't gotten to yet. Get it working right, as a whole, and the details will work themselves out. Not always but most of the time. So . . . you can now forget most of what you just learned *except this*: Remember how intricate it all is. And bear that in mind later when Jeremy tells you how important it is to do the exercises just right. Doing them wrong is literally worse than not doing them at all. Listen closely to Jeremy.

## The Muscles That Support the Spine

Interestingly, it is the *muscles* of your core—the critical spinal support system—that do the most to make your spine work correctly. Think of the core as all of the muscles between your shoulders and hips, all the way around your body: front, back, and sides. The core is the area over which you have the most control and for which you bear the most responsibility. Okay, posture, too, but tending your core is your most serious responsibility. And the most work (read "exercise").

Let's start with the muscles in the back. Close to the spine you have small muscles called "paraspinals" (in the picture below but not on the test) that act to stabilize the spine locally, preventing excessive movement, at each level, and also relaying information to the brain that tells the brain where the spine is in space. If these little guys become overloaded, they can cause painful spasms leading to debilitating pain. *Tip*: The paraspinals do in fact get overloaded all the time. Because your lousy posture puts some of your biggest and most important muscles (e.g., the glutes, in your butt) to sleep. It is one

**Paraspinal Muscles**

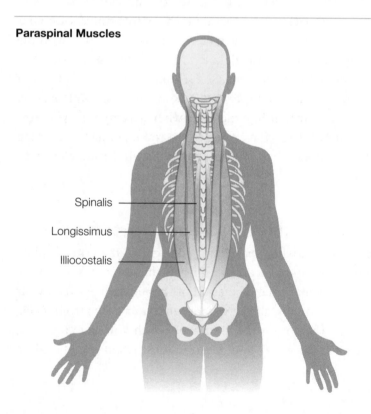

Spinalis

Longissimus

Illiocostalis

of the worst things we do to ourselves, with bad posture, idleness, and so on. Because, when the big boys fall asleep, all your weight shifts to the little guys, the paraspinals. Which fail. *Then* all that pressure goes straight onto your spine (the bones and discs), which is not designed to bear it. And all hell breaks loose. Details to follow. For now, worry about the poor little paraspinals that are going to be recruited, like child-soldiers, in a hopeless war.

Next, the body has layer upon layer of muscles, building outward (as seen in the picture on page 38), with the deepest ones labeled on the right and most superficial (nearest the skin) labeled on the left. Quite an array, isn't it? Think there's a reason

**Psoas Muscles**

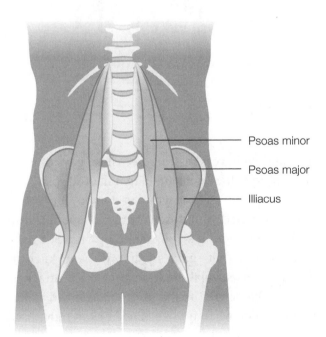

Psoas minor

Psoas major

Illiacus

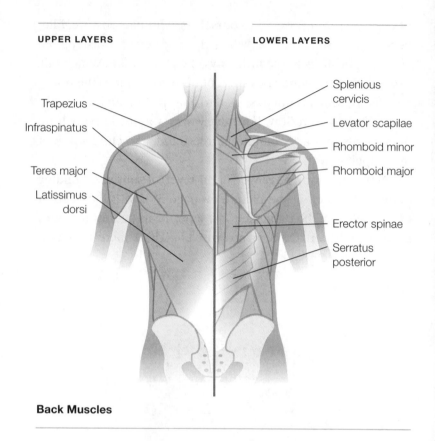

**UPPER LAYERS**

**LOWER LAYERS**

Trapezius

Infraspinatus

Teres major

Latissimus
dorsi

Splenious
cervicis

Levator scapilae

Rhomboid minor

Rhomboid major

Erector spinae

Serratus
posterior

**Back Muscles**

for that? Well, yes. Yes, there is. These guys do as much as any element to help you maintain that neutral spine.

One big muscle in your abdomen gets special mention here. It's called your "psoas" muscle (see illustration on preceding page) and it's your main hip "flexor," meaning that it is the muscle that enables you to lift your knees toward your waist. It gets special mention because it attaches directly to your lumbar spine (on the front) and can wreak havoc on your lumbar spine when it's shortened or too tight. It gets that way

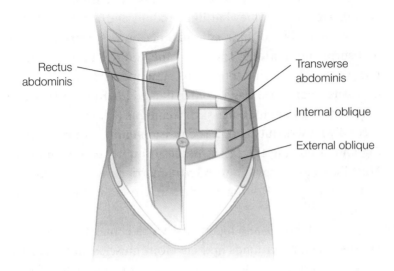

Rectus abdominis

Transverse abdominis

Internal oblique

External oblique

**Abdominal Muscles**

from prolonged sitting, or from sleeping in a fetal position. Ever wake up and feel hunched forward when you get out of bed? If you sleep in the fetal position, it might be a tight psoas you're feeling.

A lot of the muscles on our back are "extensors." That is, they are concerned with bending backward and maintaining posture. The muscles in the preceding diagram are named, but all you need to know is that they help us bend *and* they help us maintain erect posture.

On the front of our lower torso we have the muscles of the abdominal wall. The abdominal wall helps to create a stiff protective barrier for the spine. Used correctly (you'll learn how) it forms a girdle that braces and protects the spine from dangerous loads. See the picture above.

The last piece of the puzzle is the "fascia" tissue. Fascia is a connective tissue, somewhat like tendons and ligaments but in sheets. Some like to think of it like plastic wrap: stretchy, thin, and surprisingly strong. The next time you roast a leg of lamb, take a closer look: That tough, silvery, slippery outer layer is fascia tissue. There once was a woman named Ida Rolf who became famous for developing a massage technique ("Rolfing") that my second wife was nuts about. It consisted entirely of manipulating and stretching the fascia tissue to improve your mobility. Hurt like blazes. It was a wonderful marriage, it really was. But I have to tell you, Rolfing was no fun. Good for you, I bet, but no fun.

Unlike tendons and ligaments, which connect one piece to another, fascia surrounds and envelops muscles and other tissues. Fascia is very thin and helps transfer mechanical forces throughout the body from one muscle group to another. The upshot is that fascia tissue helps muscle and other tissues interact and glide smoothly over one another. Fascia helps connect the muscles that support the spine and allows smooth function while helping to transfer loads safely. If the fascia gets messed up, pain. Again. *Basic message: There are tons of things that can go wildly wrong and cause terrible pain, if you don't follow Jeremy's wise counsel.*

## What Goes Wrong: The Details of Pain

I have mentioned several times that this or that can go wrong and cause terrible pain. Let us take a moment to talk about the *details* of what can go wrong and cause all that pain. As I keep stressing, Jeremy sees your pain "whole" and does not get locked into the specifics. But he and I both think it's not a bad idea for you to know a little bit about the specifics—the *locus* of the pain—before he gets into his "whole-body" magic.

So, what goes wrong and where? Lots of stuff, but let's start with the "bulging disc"—the young man's problem, the young woman's problem. Take a look at the picture on the page 42. It doesn't look that bad but it is. You put pressure on the vertebrae—and the related discs—by the way you carry yourself or move, and darned if the disc doesn't "pooch out" a little. As in the picture. This is not the worst thing that can happen to you but *it hurts*. Quite a bit, sometimes. If you want to be upbeat about it, you can say this is Mother Nature's way of warning you that you're doing some stuff wrong and you'd better change.

Step two on the road to agony is much, much worse. It is a "burst" or "herniated disc." Again, this treat is mostly for you kids (age thirty plus). At this point, the bulge in the disc pops. The goo inside spills out and runs all over the place. Which is quite an intense experience because it frequently hits a nerve root and causes ferocious pain down the path of the nerve. How come? There are two main causes: mechanical and chemical irritation. Mechanical irritation is caused when a piece of the herniated disc compresses the nerve. This can cause pain, loss of sensation, and in more serious cases, loss of muscle function. Even when there is no physical compression of the nerve root you can have pain caused by chemical irritation of the nerve root. This happens when inflammatory chemicals are released after damage to the disc, which then irritate the nerve, causing pain along the path of the nerve. In the next picture on page 42, you get a peek at a herniated disc and a displaced and compressed nerve. You truly don't want that. Hurts a ton. You may get "radicular pain," which is the kind that shoots down your leg. Bad. As Jeremy will explain, radicular pain may mean you want to get to a medical doctor pretty damn soon, because this book alone is not going to cure you. Not soon enough, anyway. Radicular pain is bad.

Here's some other bad stuff, and now it's time for the grown-ups to take their beating. It is pain caused by general shrinking. Little old guys, little old ladies (and some who are not so old) get shorter as they age. I have had that experience (I lost about an inch and hated it). I was 5'11" to begin with (that's still what it says on my driver's license; along with "red" hair). And now I am 5'10", on a clear day. Awful! As we hinted in the introduction, the cause of this unpleasantness is "compression," especially compression of your spine. And more especially your discs. Time and gravity have had their way with you and pressed the vertebrae down. Makes sense when you think about it but it's still bad. You lose height mostly because you lose *disc height*. The vertebrae press down, the doughnuts shrink, and you get shorter. By the way, being a good kid and working out and having good posture,

**Disc Damage**

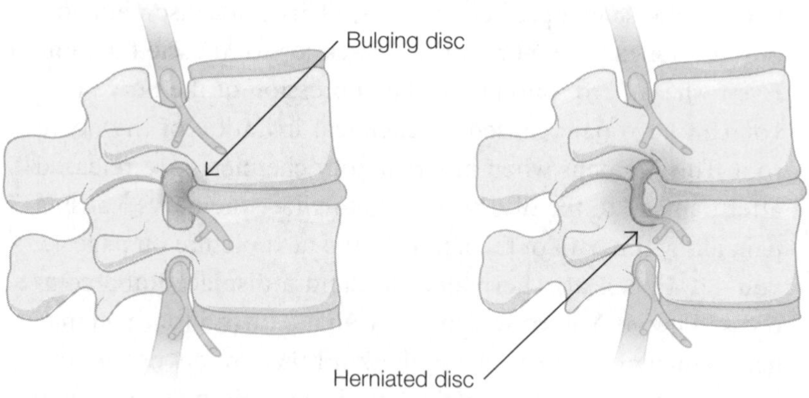

Bulging disc

Herniated disc

and so on, will *not* save you from shrinking; it's just part of aging. Sorry. Of course, you can make it a lot worse by being a dope, but you're going to have some of it regardless.

When you lose disc height, things get a little crowded along your spine—already a pretty crowded environment—and the vertebral segments don't move as they should. Lots of things can start to go wrong. Makes sense: The "washer" that's separating the bones doesn't work as well anymore. For example, the facet joints (remember them?) bump into other bone bits and become arthritic. Which is to say, "inflamed" and sore. (That's one of the things you make worse by eating like a little pig and increasing inflammation.) They get inflamed mostly because of the wear and tear on the cartilage-lined parts of those joints. In a variation on this nastiness, unhealthy stress can be placed on the discs themselves because of problems with the facet joints or another part of the spine. (Remember, it was always crowded down there, and now it's getting more so.) The picture on page 44 shows a lot of things going to hell. Note that the "inflamed joint" is a facet joint. I told you that those little suckers could cause problems.

Other aspects of you getting shorter, in the same illustration, are bone spurs and "thinned discs." How come and what do they do? I don't know, but apparently it's not good. So watch it.

This next bit sounds particularly scary to me: "central spinal stenosis." Stenosis is the narrowing of the spinal column. It is caused by all kinds of things, including simple wear and tear over time (we are talking the body's version of geologic time . . . decades of your life). Narrowing may be caused by bone spurs, disc bulges, or some misalignment of the vertebrae. You will recall that your precious spinal cord (the great bundle of nerves that runs your whole life) goes trundling down that canal. Giving it less room to do that is not a great idea.

## A Little Preview of Salvation

You're not going to be able to do much to prevent spinal stenosis, but you can do something. What you *can do*—and it makes all the difference—is to conduct your life (which is to say, maintain good posture and basic movement patterns) in such a way as to get the most out of your narrowed spinal canal. And *the great news is* that there is a lot of *redundancy and extra room* built into the system. What I mean is that there are so many joints, ligaments, muscles, tendons, and so on in the spine that just because one part is wrecked doesn't mean you are toast. Unlike the knee, hip, elbow, and other joints, there are ways to learn to be completely functional and pain-free even if a joint in your back looks god-awful on an X-ray or MRI. You can use the muscles to stabilize the problematic segment and move with other parts. Not true in other joints. So your back will work just fine, if you do some key stuff, like carrying yourself correctly. You're still gonna

**Age-Related Damage**

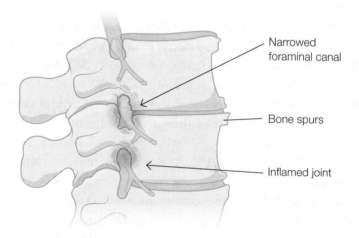

Narrowed foraminal canal

Bone spurs

Inflamed joint

be a bit shorter, though. Awful sorry about that. I begged Jeremy to say there was some way to reverse that. He said, "No!" Just like that, "No!" Sigh! I *hate being* shorter.

## More Bad News

This nasty pressure on the spine because of gravity and aging also attacks the "holes" where the major nerves exit the spinal column. The cute name for this unpleasantness is "foraminal

**Stenosis**

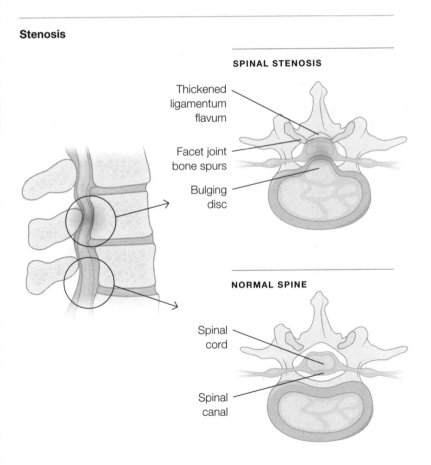

SPINAL STENOSIS

Thickened ligamentum flavum

Facet joint bone spurs

Bulging disc

NORMAL SPINE

Spinal cord

Spinal canal

stenosis." Those little holes where the nerves come out are called the foramina, and the problem is the narrowing of those holes. The compression impinges on the nerves, and, sure enough, they hurt. But, again, the good news is that sound behavior, good posture, and a powerful core can offset all that. Even after the holes are compressed, they are big enough for the nerve to pass uncompromised. If you carry yourself correctly and otherwise do exactly what Jeremy says. Otherwise, you're doomed.

By the way, does it cross your mind, as you look closely at the picture on page 44, that the narrowing of the dreaded foraminal canal would be quite a lot worse if your back were arched so as to put all the pressure on the edge that's hurting? You bet it would. That's just one of those things for you to start thinking about, as you go deeper into the book. Stand up *straight*! Think *neutral spine*! That's the stuff.

That's the walk down the spine, You don't have to *know* all this cold; it's just background for what Jeremy's going to teach you.

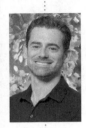

## CHAPTER FOUR

# The Spectrum of Pain: Four Patients

**From Jeremy**

You've read the story of my back pain. Maybe it sounded familiar (I hope not; it was a bear). In any event, read the next four case histories, because one of them is likely to remind you a lot of yourself. The idea is for you to see where you fit on the spectrum of back pain problems.

## Fit Fred

A lot of my Aspen-based patients are fit, knowledgeable, and a little surprised to find themselves in need of professional help for back pain. A recent patient, call him Fit Fred, is typical. He is fifty-five years old, a nice guy, in good shape, and smart. He has had serious back pain for six months. In his case, that means a bothersome ache in his lower back almost all the time. *And* intermittent periods of excruciating pain, once every two weeks or so. Those interludes—which have happened more often recently—last from a few minutes to more than an hour. It is those intervals that have driven him to seek treatment.

I am not his first stop. He's tried traditional chiropractic doctors, physical therapy, massage, and Rolfing. His back pain gets a little better for a time, and then comes back full force. When the pain is at its worst, he's stuck in bed or on the floor. He has tried traditional medicine, too, and his doctor is asking him to consider surgery. He has come to me first, because he has heard how often back surgery does not work, and he dreads that option, but he's getting closer to taking it.

"My doctor says I have degenerative disc disease. He says I have the MRI of an eighty-year-old!" (It is almost a comfort to him to think that he had "degenerative disc disease" and that an operation may fix it. He's had enough. He's giving the nonmedical approach one more chance. Then it's the knife.)

In reality, "degenerative disc disease" is a term used to describe a host of changes in the spine as a result of, or in addition to, a loss of disc height (compression) over time. As a diagnostic matter, saying that someone has degenerative disc disease doesn't amount to an awful lot more than saying that he or she is getting a little older and that his or her back hurts. That sounds a little snide, I'm afraid, but it's true. Because Fred seems to have decent posture and is in pretty good shape, I suspect that his problem is going to be related to the normal degenerative changes of the spine that go with aging and bad repetitive motions. Maybe golf, maybe yoga. Depending on how open he is to change, this could be a comparatively easy case.

It won't *sound* easy, if I go into the details. After all, compression of the spine through normal aging does do some serious things. They can include arthritic changes in the facet joints (remember them?), loss of cartilage around all the joints, foraminal stenosis, which—you will recall—is a narrowing of the opening, or foramen, from which the nerve roots exit the spine. It may be spondylolisthesis, which is a slippage of one vertebra over another, causing pain and instability—and is almost as nasty as it is unpronounceable. That all sounds awful, but they are normal concomitants of aging and degeneration of the spine and bad movements—my normal material. Those we can fix.

As for his eighty-year-old's MRI, it probably does look pretty grim. But I have to tell you, almost all MRIs of people over forty look terrible. Stuff happens, and the individual manifestations look very scary. But they are not really all that bad. Which is why I rarely prescribe MRIs unless there are signs of the scary stuff (cancer, infection, fracture, etc.); they don't tell me anything I don't already know. "Hey, you're getting older, your back is getting squished. What did you expect?" It's more sophisticated than that, but that's a fair summary in most cases. It is also a fair description of a condition you and I can fix, with behavioral change and hard work.

I ask Fred a couple of questions about the therapy he's had so far. The chiropractor has just been manipulating him with no mention of exercise. I *know* that's not going to work for a permanent fix. And the physical therapist does not seem to have much of a plan: He has had my new patient do four exercises for three months—always the same four, over and over, with no supervision and no progression. And neither of them has discussed his other activities (sports, work, exercises, etc.) with him. Beyond that, they are not the kind of exercises I will suggest because, among other things, they have done nothing to affect the endurance of the muscles of the core. This is by no means a slight on all chiropractors or physical therapists. There are some great ones out there. Some practice the way Fred's did, and some don't. Later in the book, we give you some pointers on finding good ones.

Fred really is active, God bless him, but he's doing some activities that, I suspect, are not helping his back. He does quite a lot of yoga, plays golf regularly, and lifts weights in the gym. A very responsible, fit guy, as I say. But what I know, without seeing him do yoga or play golf, is that some of the movements in those two activities are often a source of serious back injury over time. There is a safe, spine-healthy way to do yoga but, done wrong, as it often is, it can cause terrible problems. For now, I tell him to lay off yoga completely for at least two months. He can get back to it in time with some modifications. The same with golf. Golf is a wonderful activity. Not great exercise (contrary to what so many insist) but a wonderful way to be with friends and go to beautiful places. It can also be, structurally, one of the worst things you can do to your back. (All that one-way twisting of your lumbar spine.) There is a spine-healthy way to play golf, but for now I just tell him to lay off the golf until he is educated enough to be open to some instruction on a "right way" to play. [Hint: You learn to rotate with your *hips* more at the end of your swing, and less with your lower back.]

Then I asked him to walk me through his strength-training regimen. It was not the worst strength regimen I have ever heard about, but it was pretty bad. He was doing a number of things that were *almost criminally bad* for him. If *you* are doing a lot of strength training, there is a sad chance that you, too, are doing some seriously harmful stuff, from a back point of view. That's because we were *all trained* to do things wrong, back in the day.

Take, for example, the traditional "army sit-up," which Fred is still doing. We all did a lot of those at one point and a lot of us are doing them still. Even the army gave them up only in recent times. But the fact is that there are few things worse for your back than the good old army sit-up. (A shallow, or four-inch "crunch" is fine, and it does all you need for your core; you do not need to bend your spine like a pretzel to get a benefit.)

The sit-up, where you twist to touch your elbow to the opposite knee, is the worst of all. And that's just one of a bunch of deeply familiar exercises that are fundamentally terrible for your back. The machines we all used to love are a particular peril (not all but many). The whole world of bad strength training makes me particularly crazy: Here are these terrific men and women, working so hard in an effort to make their bodies stronger and better. And what they are doing is, in fact, worse than doing nothing at all. Sad and wrong.

Most important, Fit Fred has no notion of the importance of engaging his core and strengthening his core and glutes—perhaps the most important elements in a sane strength-training regimen. And he doesn't have a clue about the importance of decent posture and of maintaining a neutral spine. So I tell him to stop all strength training until I can show him how to do it right.

## Substantial Sally

If Fit Fred was on the fit end of the fitness spectrum, then Substantial Sally was the opposite. She is *significantly* overweight (she is close to 300 pounds, which is very significant indeed) and has had no regular exercise program for the past four years. She has had a whopping four spine surgeries, two in the past two years, including a fusion and a laminectomy. Fusions are common, but they are very serious business indeed. It is a procedure in which the surgeon uses hardware to *bolt (fuse)* two or more vertebrae together to prevent further movement at that joint. There is a place for fusions, but I see them as a very last resort. They give relief, but if the person does not make the necessary behavioral changes, they often find themselves having *another fusion* or other problems in a few years. They are not a *cure*, in any broad sense. A laminectomy is a less serious procedure in which the surgeon removes a small piece of bone off a vertebra to relieve pressure on a particular nerve. Again, it cures a symptom, not the basic problem.

In any event, Sally has been through the wars, she is still in pain, and she is both smart and wary. She is not one bit sure that I am going to be any more help than my predecessors. I don't blame her. But I think she's wrong. I think I am going to be able to help her quite a lot, if she'll listen, which she may not.

Sally is an appealing woman, the head of a company that she started herself, and which she has made a huge success of. I automatically like her, right off; she's one of those people whom everyone likes right off . . . part of her success, I assume. But she sure is in trouble, and it is making her cranky. I don't blame her, but she is not fun. Not many of my patients are fun; they hurt too much.

Sally's basic problem, in my view, is behavioral. That is, she has not been taking care of herself while she has been taking care of business. She has put on a ton of weight, to begin with, which hasn't helped. And she has had a lot of pain. Interestingly (and familiarly to me), the fear of its onset has been almost as bad as the pain itself. That hasn't helped her business either, she says. Like Fit Fred, she reads off the list of things her medical doctor says are wrong with her with something approaching pride. And, sure enough, the list goes on for quite a while. She has central stenosis, foraminal stenosis (that's what the second operation was for, but it's back), bone spurs (bony growths like calluses, but on the bone), and good old spondylolisthesis (a slippage of one vertebra over another, which hurts).

Of the *four* surgeries she has had, the most recent two, the fusion and the laminectomy, relieved some of her debilitating leg and foot pain for a while, but serious back pain remains, along with intermittent bouts of buttock and leg pain when she walks. We talk about her postsurgical physical therapy. It helped somewhat while she was doing it but the lower back pain always came back. Now everything she does hurts. Walking, sitting, standing, you name it. She scoffs when I ask about resuming an exercise regimen. "That, sir, is impossible." Well, we'll see.

I start by asking her to get up on the table and lie on her back. Not so fast, she says. That is almost beyond her. She weighs an awful lot and every move hurts. It is not easy for her to get on the table, and she doesn't like it. I help her, but I weigh only about 150; I can see her thinking to herself, "Maybe a bigger therapist?" But we get there. Once she settles into the position on her back, I ask her to bend her knees and put her feet flat on the table. *Same thing I told myself to do, that day of my back spasm.* It hurts, she says. I ignore that, and tell her to move her legs up and down as if marching in place, bringing the knees up toward the torso. Does this make your back hurt? Of course it does. But—sneaky, I know—she is getting used to the idea that *I* think it's going to be possible for her to move in this position, which is true. Okay, I say, let's lessen the range of motion a lot. Now just barely lift your feet off of the table. Does this make your back hurt? Yes. Growing frustration.

Now I shift gears and, for the next fifteen minutes, I talk to her about finding her neutral spine. She does. Then I ask her to tighten the muscles in her abdomen, which—God bless her— she finally does. I'm getting off track and talking a bit about the beginning of therapy, I know, but therapy and diagnosis are inseparable in her case.

Then I have her do the marching in place again, but with those muscles engaged. Does that hurt? "No," she says with surprise. And darned if she doesn't brighten a little. A wisp of pleasure or relief comes across her face. Huh!

I tell her that she has just crossed the Rubicon. We have begun on the road to a cure. It is going to be long and hard, but my guess is that we are going to get there. "Yeah?" she asks, not daring to believe it.

"Yeah," I say, "I believe we are. No guarantees and a lot of work for you. But my guess is that you've been a worker all your life, that you'll work at this and that you will make it. Yes." She is plenty skeptical, but she smiles, too.

I explain that if she can move her legs without pain in her back while lying down then she can eventually do it upright. And that is called walking. It has been a while since she was able to walk without pain, and there have been plenty of days when she couldn't walk at all. I push her to do a little more, but that little march is all she can do for now. Fine, that's where we start.

There can be a serious, psychological component in all this, and it was very serious indeed with Sally. She had become deeply scared of movement. Any and all movement because any movement hurts. Her default solution has been not to move at all. Worse than that, her real solution in recent times has been to sit on the sofa and drink quite a bit of white wine. It worked, in a way, but was disastrous, too. It has given her this hideous weight problem. It hasn't made her very good company, and it has been brutal for her business. But she didn't hurt when doing that. So she sat on the couch for many hours a day, doing some business and quite a lot of drinking. My complicated task—and the book may not be much help on this one—was to wean her from the sofa-and-wine solution and get her into the *movement* solution. I was cautiously optimistic. Justifiably optimistic, it turns out. She is a proud woman and had a right to be. I thought that that fact and the early easing of pain just might do the job.

## THE GATEWAY THEORY OF PAIN

**H**ere is a little anecdote about the walking-in-place solution with which so many cures begin. A big reason for the reduction of pain is that tensing the abdominal muscles in the right way keeps the spine from moving and causing irritation. But, another reason is that it is a simple distraction from pain, to get the patient to focus on movement. We have gateways or pathways over which pain moves to the brain, and they have a limited capacity. One of the things about the walking-in-place phenomenon is that the "reports" of this activity to the brain take up a fair amount of neural space and *block the gateways.* There is less room for the pain reports to get through. So they don't. Some do, of course, but fewer. Thus, the simple business of walking-in-place, which serves many functions, blocks the pain highway and lessens the sense of pain. Sounds trifling but it works. It's like the nurse pinching the spot where she's going to give you the shot: she wants to keep you busy. Your neural pathways, anyway.

Sally and I have been at it for six months and she has done remarkably well. We are not there yet, but she has made terrific progress, her spirits are much improved, and her drinking much abated. Six months into our work, she is walking with her spouse around the neighborhood at night without much pain. She is playing with her grandchildren. She is going to the movies. She goes to the office rather than having everything brought to her at home. And she is doing serious (for her) strength training! She sees all this as a near-miracle and is charmingly grateful. Is she totally pain-free? No. She may never be. Does she have her life back? Yes, quite a bit of it, anyway. I want to see her make more progress. She thinks what has happened thus far is extraordinary.

## Regular Robert

On the fitness scale, Regular Robert was somewhere in the middle. In terms of his lifestyle and temperament, he was a lunatic. Like a lot of my patients here in Aspen, he is successful, a strong alpha personality, a serious workaholic, and a handful. He *thinks* he's a fitness guy but his idea of fitness is getting on the treadmill for forty-five minutes a day while reading his emails. This is not my idea of fitness; this is my idea of fooling around. And it is largely useless for someone with real back issues. The rest of his day is spent in intense meetings, traveling, and (especially) bent over his computer. Recently, he has had a relatively sudden onset of pretty serious lower back and buttock pain. It is nowhere near as severe as what I had or what most of the other people in this chapter had, but it's serious enough, and he's not liking it one bit. So here he sits, in my office, looking cranky. Everyone I see looks cranky.

I listen to his story and determine it is likely a bulging lumbar disc. Do you remember those terms? *Lumbar* means lower back, where almost all back pain resides. And a disc is a disc. The reasons behind my conclusion are fairly straightforward *and* you can probably follow the analysis yourself, if you have similar problems. By asking him to move some, I find that he gets more pain with *flexion* (forward bending at the waist), sitting, and lifting. The pain eases with standing, *extension* (backward bending at the waist), and moving. The pain radiates down into his buttocks and can go from severe to almost nonexistent in the same day. The pain is more severe in the back than in the buttock or leg. I believe that it is a *bulge* (the outer fibers of the disc are still mostly intact) and not a *herniation* or rupture because the pain would be more severe if it were a rupture, and it would likely be radiating down his leg.

The pain is positional, meaning it gets better or worse depending on the position he is in. The pain goes from fairly intense to fairly mild, sometimes within hours, and he is not complaining of any numbness in his leg or foot. When the disc is herniated, it is common for the pain to be constant regardless of position and there is apt to be accompanying numbness or tingling in the foot or leg. The pain is also commonly the most intense in the leg or foot and not the back. I tell him I think he has a bulging disc and I explain just what that means. Type A guy that he is, he immediately wants to talk about surgery—about getting this *fixed*! Right now. "How bad is the surgery? How long is the recovery?" he asks. "Who should I use and how soon can I schedule it?"

I tell him to chill for a minute; we are nowhere near that point yet. There are various stages of disc dysfunction, I tell him, and his does not look that bad to me. I say this because my exam shows no neurological damage. Here's what I mean. I tapped his Achilles tendon and his foot jerked sharply, a sign that there has been no nerve damage in that area. I do the same with his knee (the same spot your doctor taps when you have a physical): same result. His reflexes are normal, so likely no nerve damage. His strength is within normal range, too.

If you have even a hint of "radicular" pain—pain that goes down your leg—you should see a medical doctor. It could be pain from an irritated nerve root (which can be serious) or it could be referred muscular pain. The analysis is a bit too complicated to cover in a book. In any event, I conclude that Regular Robert has not suffered any motor nerve damage because of nerve compression and he has not suffered any loss of strength. In the absence of serious motor function or nerve loss, surgery is seldom called for.

Let me repeat this: Self-assessment gets tricky when it comes to muscle and nerve loss. If you sense that you are anywhere near that territory, especially if you have possible radicular pain (pain going down your leg), you should get professional help, probably a medical doctor.

Regular Robert does not have nerve or muscle loss so he is not likely to have suffered a herniation. He is lucky, in a way, to have come in with this problem at this stage. It will give him a not-so-gentle kick in the pants to take spine health seriously. And it will give me a chance to offer him major relief, if not an outright cure. *If* he is serious and does what he must.

In the short term, I give him instructions similar to what I have told the others. I tell him to stop doing some things and start doing others. I tell him to keep up the aerobic exercise but do not expect it alone to do much for his back. I tell him urgently that he has to give up sitting for such long stretches. He, incidentally, sits on a giant ball and assumes that makes all the difference; it doesn't. It only helps if it makes you get up and move about more often, which it may or may not do.

The trick with sitting is to *do much less of it.* And to get up and vary your position frequently. Sitting puts more pressure on the lumbar discs than any other position. Much more. It's too bad but we just were not designed for it. So stand up every thirty minutes or so, and move around. The great trick is to mix it up. After that, the big change in his life is going to be a serious and very different exercise regimen, to build up his core and support his back. He is going to be a success story; I can just feel it.

## Doomed Daniel

Doomed Daniel had symptoms that I thought made him a candidate for surgery, not just behavioral change. You'll want to read his story closely, not because you are likely to be in the same boat—that is actually very unlikely—but because, if you are, you should know about it, and you'll want to act expeditiously. As you'll see, Daniel insisted on going down the behavioral change road for quite a long time, and it did not hurt him. But you may want to move a little more promptly. Just to be crystal clear, if you sound like Daniel, then this book is not for you. Not for now, anyway. If you have surgery, you may very well want to come back to the book later, since surgery does not routinely provide a permanent cure without necessary behavioral change.

Daniel is thirty-five, an avid outdoorsman, and he comes in with excruciating pain, pain shooting down his leg to the ankle. *Radicular pain*, as you now know. His periodic back spasms can last hours or days. The pain comes on suddenly after he's been exercising—snowmobiling, in his most recent case. After the initial spasm, the pain gets worse every day. He describes a shocking or burning sensation, which he rates as a 9/10 in severity. He has had mild lower back pain for over a year, before this new problem began.

The lower back pain was achy and annoying for a long time, but not enough to bring him to a doctor. The new pain is something else entirely. I examine him and note that he has mild foot drop (a weakening of the muscles that flex the ankles). I note this because he is unable to walk across the room on his heels; his affected foot will not stay up while he walks. This is indicative of nerve damage. He also has a loss of sensation in various parts of his leg in a dermatomal pattern, which also points to the likelihood of nerve damage. But, just for the record, dermatomal patterns mean that the pattern of sensation loss is a predictable pattern of the kind that arises from injury to a particular vertebra or disc. It's kind of interesting: Each nerve and nerve root supplies sensation to specific areas of your body. You can therefore map them out in a reliable, predictable way. If you see "drop foot" with numbness along the top of the foot, you can reasonably suggest that the L5 nerve root is compressed and that there is likely a disc herniation at the L5/S1 disc. Is that confusing? Fine, forget about it; you don't need to know.

Taken together, those things—the radicular pain shooting down his leg and the loss of nerve function manifested by the insensitivity to touch and the "dropped foot"—strongly suggest that this is not just a bulging disc but actually a ruptured or "herniated" disc. That means that the disc has broken and the goo inside is running all over the place. The year of an achy lower back was a *bulging* disc. But the pain shooting down the leg and the nerve damage suggest that the disc has popped, presumably when he landed on his snowmobile off of a big jump. He'd been building up to this for a long time. Now it's probably time for surgery.

Unlike a lot of people, Daniel is absolutely determined *not* to have surgery and to resolve the problem with exercise and hard work. I sympathize but tell him, with regret, that I doubt very much that it will work. He still insists. I say, fine, if you can stand the pain, I will start therapy. Which we did.

But, as I expected, it's just too hard. As an interim step, just because he is so determined not to have surgery, I send him to a pain doc, but I am still worried. He is risking a permanent "foot drop" and that's nuts. After a few sessions, the pain is as bad as ever, and he's now unable to sleep. He tries various pain and sleep medications but nothing works. Finally, I persuade him to see a neurosurgeon. They schedule him for surgery the following week.

I am delighted to report that the surgery was a complete success. Six weeks later, his back pain was minimal. But here is the *real* happy ending. In the course of our time together, he has come to understand that surgery, as marvelous as it can be, is a fix, not a cure. So he came back to see me four months after surgery to start some basic training to avoid finding himself in the same mess, a year or two from now. He takes it all seriously. He will not find himself back in surgery.

## Are You in "The 20 Percent"?

Daniel was in the 20 percent I could not help, at least not in the first instance. His condition had proceeded so far that he needed conventional medical help, and he needed it urgently. So, how do you establish whether you are in the 20 percent who should seek medical help?

Before turning to that, here is some general advice for all of you. There is a small, a very small, possibility that just about any back pain may be a marker for cancer. The risk is remote, but the downside is big, so I urge all my back pain patients to go to a regular medical doctor before they do anything else, just to check out that possibility.

For other conventional reasons to seek regular medical help, there are some reliable indications.

1. If you have lower back pain with *numbness* in the buttocks, leg, or foot, you need to be evaluated by a physician to monitor for potential nerve damage. Once that issue is disposed of, by all means come back to the book for further help.

2. If you have lower back pain and are exhibiting *signs of muscle loss*, such as dragging your foot, "foot drop," tripping, etc, you need to see a regular doc. Loss of muscle strength is a sign of nerve damage, which can be irreversible. You need to see a physician *immediately*. Depending on how that goes, you may again want to come back to the book for more comprehensive care.

3. In the same vein, if you have lower back pain with tingling in the buttock or leg, you need to see a physician to monitor potential nerve damage.

4. If you have severe lower back pain that never varies in intensity and does not seem to be related to movement, activity, or position, you need to see a physician at once. Your back pain may be caused something other than musculoskeletal issues.

5. If you have radicular pain that shoots down your leg, often past your knee to your foot, and if the pain is extremely acute, see a physician. You may have ruptured a disc and should seek medical care right away. You may need surgery.

For the rest of you, this book should do the trick. And, even for those of you who should consider surgery or other medical help, there is strong likelihood that you will want to come back to the book, later on, to seek a *permanent* solution to your problem. Often, medical solutions, indispensable though they may be in certain situations, are not permanent.

## CHAPTER FIVE

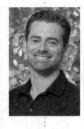

## RULE #1

# Stop Doing Dumb Stuff

**From Jeremy**

N ow we are down to the nuts and bolts of what I do for my patients in the office and what I am going to do for you in this book. For convenience, we call it the "James Protocol" or just the "Protocol"; either is fine. And to give it some structure and make it easier to follow, we have boiled it down to Seven Rules (see page 241). Think of them as seven paths to freedom from back pain, if you like, but the point is that there are seven of them and they are the main markers on your path to an end of pain.

## Rule #1: Stop Doing Dumb Stuff

I like this rule because it is so obvious. *And* so important. Virtually all of us with back pain are doing one or more dumb things that trigger that pain. Not because we are thick. I have dealt with some of the smartest people in the country, and they are as susceptible to these errors as anyone else. The problem is that we just have not been alerted to the problems. Or we have fallen into them so gradually that we never noticed.

By the way, this is not the beginning of what you might think of as the Big Fix—the fundamental changes that are going to make a permanent difference. But you cannot turn to that before you make the darned pain go away. Rule #1 is to make the pain go away by the simple step of ceasing to do the stuff that *immediately* causes it. As obvious as that sounds, an awful lot of healers and sufferers haven't latched on to this.

How do you recognize the behaviors that hurt your back or trigger back pain? From long experience, I have learned most people *know*, at some level, what they are doing wrong. Their *first* response is apt to be wrong, though. At first, they'll want to tell you about some particular incident. "I rolled over in bed funny." "I bent over to retie my shoe." "I took a long flight (or whatever)." It's interesting: Almost everyone thinks that the little event is the dreadful thing that "did it." In fact, that is rarely the case.

But their second response is better. If you dig a little, what you eventually hear about is patterns of behavior that have lasted years, decades in fact, that are almost certainly the real cause of the pain. The most obvious one, which we come back to again and again because it is so important to so many: "I've been curled up over my computer a lot lately." Another popular one: "It crops up after I play golf (tennis, bowling, or whatever)." Or: "It's worse after strength training." Or yoga, or whatever. So, it is not moving "funny" one time in the night. It is moving funny—often in the same way—for decades. Which makes it more obvious, when you think about it. And a bit more difficult to change.

I listen carefully to these stories and I am very interested indeed in these particular causes. But I confess that I have been at this so long and have known "the enemy" for so long that I take what may seem like a surprisingly broad-brush approach. I *know* the behaviors that have caused the greatest problems for almost all my patients and I now take the simple approach of telling everyone to stop *all of them*. At least in the first instance. There will be time to sort out particular problems (and get you back into particular activities) later on. But for now, I urge you to stop doing all the following:

- Sitting for hours at your computer (details to follow)
- Yoga
- Downhill skiing or snowboarding
- All strength training (whether with weights or not)
- Golf
- Snowmobiling
- Tennis or other racquet sports
- Uphill hiking
- Pilates (yes, Pilates)
- Horseback riding
- Running
- Cycling
- Prolonged sitting—in the car, a plane, or wherever.
- Anything else that involves bending, twisting, pounding, or otherwise pressuring your back

You may be shocked by this list but don't worry. We'll have you back to most of these activities pretty soon. And back to all of them, eventually, but with modified movements that don't hurt your back. Admittedly, this is a pretty serious first step, but back pain is a pretty serious affliction, as you know.

## SITTING FOR HOURS AT YOUR COMPUTER

The most serious of these "stop being dumb" problems—and the hardest to address—is sitting for hours at your computer. You will say you simply *can't* stop that. It's your job, it's what you do for a living, it's your life, and so on. All right, I surely understand that: It's what slapped me on my back, in agony, not too long ago. Working at the computer was my life, too, but it almost put an end to my career.

So let's address that one first, the irresistible business of sitting for hours at your computer. The first fix—and it won't be easy at first—is just to get up every twenty or thirty minutes and move around. That alone will do wonders. Do that religiously, and you can continue to use your computer.

Folks tell me that they cannot get up that often. They will lose their train of thought, they will get jumpy and weird . . . they just can't do it. Well, yes, they can. And they have to, because continuing to do what you do is not working for you. So just plain do it. Get up. Change your position. Do some stretches. Go chat with someone. Do anything. In my experience, your concentration will be better, not worse, once you get slightly used to it. Whether or not that turns out to be true for you, just do it. It is a critical first step for many, many of you.

## SOME OTHER TRICKS

It may help to get a standing desk. But please bear in mind that it is not the standing that is the answer, it's the movement. You are more apt to move around if you work at a standing desk, which is good. But make no mistake: It is just as bad to stand in one position all day as to sit in one position all day. *Movement and change* are the answers, not buying a standing desk. Some people get so serious about this that they buy "treadmill desks," so you are actually walking (very slowly) as you work. I haven't tried it.

The same goes for sitting on a big exercise ball. That, per se, doesn't do much good (indeed, your posture may get worse, which is disastrous). But you are more likely to move, on the ball. Try it if it appeals to you.

The most obvious (and effective) thing to do is to just get up and walk around for a moment or two, every half hour or so. Another solution, just change *the way* you're sitting from time to time. I hate to say this but, if your posture is pretty good, hunch forward for a few minutes, once in a while. Be "bad." If your posture is lousy, by all means make it good, and use good posture most of the time. But any movement is good, including the occasional slouch. It's movement that matters, any movement. Cross your knees, from time to time. Hold your legs out straight and tense your muscles as hard as you can, and hold for 20 seconds. It feels good and it works. Lean back, opening up the front of your hip, bend forward without rounding your back. Jiggle one foot. Any silly excuse to move will do. But move.

Why is movement so critical? Because it is an answer to "creep," and creep is serious business.

## Creep

*Creep* sounds bad, and it is. Creep refers to the fact that your body can actually become *deformed* in a surprisingly short time, by your rotten (static) behavior. Put parts of your body under stresses that they were not designed to bear for a stretch of time, and a bad thing happens: They deform. If you subject the tissues in your back to "static flexion," from prolonged sitting, the tissues in your back start to deform and stretch, causing instability in the spine. This puts the harmful loads directly through the discs and joints. The same with "repetitive flexion," which means bending over again and again, at some repetitive task. (Think gardening, or improper weightlifting.) Again, the muscles and other tissues that normally protect the spine become lax and deformed, causing immediate pain and long-term damage. This also sets you up for potential disaster when you stand. Your spine is now unstable and subject to serious damage if you were to lift something heavy before the tissues return to their normal state. This can have even more serious, permanent results. That's creep, and it is not good.

Think how your body behaves in noncreep mode. When we are in good posture, that is. When you maintain a neutral spine (we'll get into the details of this critical concept in a moment), the muscles, tendons, ligaments, and joint capsules in and around your spine are all rigid and taut and in balance. They hold you up. They supply stability and support to your spine and keep it neutral. It is a big deal and quite complicated. The muscles supporting the spine, especially the little ones in and around your vertebrae called "multifidi," have lots of *mechanoreceptors* (little sensory organs) that respond to physical, mechanical stimuli such as touch or load. Those little ones help us maintain a safe spinal position via *reflexes*. Not the big reflexes like the one that jerks your leg when the doc taps your knee in a certain place. Little guys that do the same thing on a much smaller scale. But these little guys do big work. They trigger lightning-quick changes in muscle tension and joint stiffness to allow us to make minute changes in spine position and muscle strength, preventing overload of the spine. This is going on all the time in our bodies, and it matters tremendously.

Think of creep like this. Think of an elastic band that has been stretched too far or for too long and becomes dusty, slack, and ineffectual. That happens to your muscles with creep. Also, the joints in the area become less stable as the muscles get lopsided. Finally, the nervous system, which manages those reflexes, gets hobbled, too. And the wrong signals (or no signals) are sent, which causes even more profound deformation. The whole system of small muscles and related nerves that hold the back in a good place goes to hell. And so does your back.

Creep causes pain, all on its own. That's because the little muscles around the joint sense that *something* is terribly wrong, and they spasm, in an effort to *hold* the status quo and protect unstable joint segments. Spasms hurt. Second, if you put a load on an unstable joint, it is not able to sustain that pressure, and major damage can occur such as a disc herniation or ligament sprain. That hurts, too.

Finally, creep sets you up for that "sudden" movement that you think is the cause of your back pain. Here is a good example: Think of a fireman sitting, stock-still, in the fire station for ten hours. He's in some kind of bad posture and he holds that bad posture so long that creep occurs. Now the bell goes off, he goes flying down the fire pole or whatever, and rushes out to the fire. Maybe he picks up a super-heavy hose. Or an unconscious person. His back has suffered serious creep, and it is in a terrible position to try to take on those loads. He "throws his back out"—way out. And he's apt to think that it was his strenuous movements that did it. Which, in a way, is true. But the real culprit was creep. And you do not have to sit in a fire station and then lift unconscious bodies to suffer from it. Sitting around the computer all day, followed by picking something slightly heavy off the floor, will do it. But for you as for the fireman, it was not the picking up that caused the pain. It was creep, and it happened over time. Creep can happen over a relatively short time, a long day at your desk. And it can really happen over extended periods of time. You "deform" your back, and it is not ready or able to do what it was designed to do.

## SO WHAT DO YOU DO TO AVOID CREEP?

As I said, the best thing is to get up and move all the time, every twenty or thirty minutes. That's the short-term solution. In the longer term, you will want to do some serious exercises, too, to strengthen your core. And before that, you have to learn to use a neutral spine. That's really key, but we can't talk about everything at once. We'll get there soon. In the meantime, get moving.

## Other Trigger Behaviors

Of course it is not just sedentary behavior that causes problems. Especially when combined with alternating patterns of idleness, like the behavior of that fireman. So don't just stop the idleness, stop the big triggering movements, too. Golf is a particular favorite. Let's assume, for a moment, that you lead a relatively sedentary life. Then you head out to the golf course and the basic movement is a wildly centrifugal twisting of your whole body—especially your lower back—as you swing for the fences. Is your back ready for that? No. Indeed, your lower back is *never* ready for that; it is not designed for that kind of torquing. You are going to have to learn to rotate much more with your *hips*, not your lower back. Don't worry, it works just about as well.

What about snowmobiling? And tennis? And all the others? We're not going to go through them one at a time, because it's too complex for a single book. But we assume that the picture is clear.

And it is not the entire sport or activity that causes problems; it's a few things. Think of weightlifting, for example. Weightlifting is great for you, and I hope you will do it forever. But most of us have not really learned to do it properly, and some of the things we do are disastrously bad. Think, for example, of the guy or gal you see at the gym, struggling with all their might to do bicep curls with very heavy dumbbells. If you look closely, you often see them tucking and bending their back in an attempt to lift the weights up, grunting and heaving all the way. This is disastrous for the spine. If you have to heave and move your back to lift a weight, it's too heavy. Using momentum by shoving your hips forward and bending your back is one of the worst things you can do for your lumbar spine. I could go on and on, but we cannot cover all of the terrible habits seen in the gym and sport at the very beginning. Better to get you to lay off all potentially harmful activities and get you back into them gradually, as you become wiser about how your back works. And doesn't work.

So, your life is not over. The fun stuff is not off-limits forever. It's just out of the picture for a bit while we teach you to move correctly. *Then* you can get back to virtually all the things on the list. But not this week. And maybe not for the next few months. You have to let your back heal. You have to learn some new behaviors. And you have to strengthen your core. Then it's back to your old activities with a new you. And they won't hurt anymore.

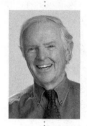

CHAPTER SIX

# Geologic Forces

......................................................................

**From Chris**

W e have talked about a lot of specifics. Now we'd like to pull the camera back a little and put all this in a broader context. The basic point, one more time: Little, very specific things go wrong with your back at specific spots — a stressed disc, a pinched nerve, a muscle spasm. But what is really going on is that huge forces are at work *on your whole body and especially on your back* that *manifest* themselves in specific ways. And the only way you're really going to heal your back and avoid long-term pain is to address these mega-forces at the root of your problems.

To open your head to the kind of thing we are talking about, think for a minute about the geologic forces that shape continents and tear mountains down to rubble. It's astonishing, really: Relatively minor pressures, like rain and wind and a succession of freezes, literally tear down mountains. It's hard to believe but undeniably true — hard to believe because those forces are so relatively trivial, compared to the strength of mountains. And yet, over time, they prevail.

So what? Well, our bodies, and especially our backs, are like that, too. Relatively minor behaviors—sitting carelessly at your computer, picking up heavy stuff with a bowed back, standing around with your head projected forward—have no impact at all, the first time. Or over a period of months, or years. Kids get away with lousy posture for a long time. But time and pressure always win. Over time—decades, say—the pressure on your back from hunching over your computer raises hell with your back. Over time, those trifling pressures from picking things up incorrectly will have you rolling on the floor. Time and pressure, "geologic pressure" on your spine, tears you down.

Once you get your head around that concept, you might think that we are all doomed, regardless of what we do—that the pressure of gravity alone, over decades, is going to wreck our backs no matter what. But here is the interesting thing: That's not true. Used correctly, your body and especially your spine are built to stand up nicely to, say, 90 or even 100 years of relentless gravity and other "geological" pressures. Stand and move correctly—which is to say, with a neutral spine—and take effective steps to keep the *core* that holds your neutral spine in place *strong*, and your back will last a hundred years. That is a slightly amazing—and hugely hopeful—thing. *Do stuff that's within your control—maintain a neutral spine, keep your core strong, and don't be stupid—and you can withstand those geological pressures for a lifetime.*

As long as we're focused on the big picture, let's recognize that we are talking about two (or more) basic types of pressure on our bodies. There's plain old gravity, which accounts for a lot. But there is also the pressure of movement. And especially regular, repetitive movement. I am talking about how we stand up or squat, how we pick things up off the floor or from the shelf. I am talking especially about the basic flexion, extension, and *rotational* movements, like when we swing around to reach something beside and below or above us. Or, say, how we serve in tennis. Or hit a golf ball. And—for you good kids who do serious strength training—how we actually pick up a set of weights, off the floor . . . do a sit-up or a plank.

And here's a basic insight: Gravity alone can raise holy hell with your back, if your posture is rotten. But the real killer is *movement*. Especially what we think of as "loaded" movement. By "loaded" we mean anything in addition to body weight, such as picking things up or lifting weights. It's bad, for example, to twist around to pick something light off the ground *if you rotate with your lower back instead of your rotating with your hips*. But if you're picking something up that weighs twenty or thirty pounds or more, the potential for harm goes up geometrically. Then add repetition and time—because you do this exercise "wrong" two days a week at the gym—then the potential for harm is enormous. Basic tip: Doing strength training "wrong" is much, much worse than not doing it at all. Some of the saddest people Jeremy, Bill, and I see—and we see them *all the time*—are older men and women who have been serious weight lifters for years who have been doing it wrong. And who now can barely move in an athletic or real-world way. And this is true even though they have biceps the size of softballs and quads that are scary. They *can't move!* Because they have been moving wrong, heavily loaded, all their lives. Their backs are a mess, as are most of their joints; the small muscles, which weight machines do not work, have atrophied. Bill and Jeremy have saved such folks, *but* it can take years of corrective exercises.

Let's look at just a few movements or postures that cause problems, and then think of them in "geologic" time. (In human terms, again, that means decades.) Take a couple of simple examples (see the illustration on this page): Look at the woman in picture A, on the left. She is picking up a substantial weight, but she has good posture, including a neutral spine. And, while you can't see it, you can assume that she has "locked down" her core to safeguard her back before she started this exercise. And her core is strong. As she rises from this position, the glutes are going to do a lot of the work, which is good. That's what they are for. The pressures of the lift are spread evenly across the various muscles of the core and the surface of her vertebrae. She can lift weights like this—assuming that she is sane about how much weight and how many reps she does—for the rest of her life and do just fine.

Now look at the poor person in picture B. She is just as well intentioned, and is picking up roughly the same amount of

**Correct and Incorrect Lifting**

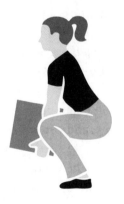

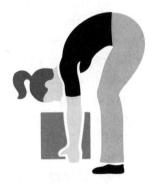

A                                    B

weight as the woman in picture A. But she is basically doomed. Because she is doing it with a bowed back. The pressures of the lift are directed through the spine and *all on the edges*. The pressure is concentrated on the edge of the disc and the vertebrae. Two things about these women. First, *the woman with the neutral spine can bear 40 percent more weight* than the other woman (assuming the two have identical strength and fitness). That's a big deal. And it's interesting: Every Olympic or otherwise serious lifter knows this and is meticulous about a neutral spine. Amateurs like you and I . . . less clear.

But the really big deal is what happens over time to the two of them. The woman who is lifting wrong (with a bowed back) is putting horrendously more pressure on the *edges* of the vertebrae and discs in her spine, and they will go bad, dramatically, in time. The other woman . . . no problem.

That was a dramatic example. But much less extreme behaviors, *repeated over a long enough time*, will have just as hellish an impact on you. Think about the basic and most common behavior, which we have talked about so much: lolling at your computer. That does not put nearly as much bad pressure on your back as weightlifting incorrectly. But *time* is a fine stand-in for weight. Do this behavior over a long span of time—as you now know—and you will make just as bad a mess of your back as bad lifting. Think, again, of geologic pressure. Gentle rains take longer to erode than hurricanes. But eventually the pressures are the same, and the mountain will come down. It's the same with you: Do dumb stuff long enough, and you will be rolling on the floor. Awful.

Do you have to be an idiot to engage in behaviors that get you in a jam? Obviously not. *All* of us sit carelessly at our computers more than we should. Including—in one embarrassing case I personally know about—a back-care professional whose initials are J-e-r-e-m-y J-a-m-e-s! And bear in mind that there are other bad "behaviors" so subtle that no one is going to focus on them. Think about this one: You have a touch of arthritis in one foot and it hurts, ever so slightly, at every step. Without even thinking about it you make a tiny adjustment in the way you walk, and it helps a lot. Trouble is, that tiny change also included a tiny change in the way you work your hip, and *that* little change was serious. You start to walk slightly differently, and now you are putting unhealthy stresses through your lower back. This is *one of the* most common ways to get your back misaligned, other than bad posture. Over time—over geologic time—that heedless adjustment of your foot and then your hip is going to bring you down. And you most assuredly didn't have to be a dope to wind up in that mess. There are hundreds of variations on that story, many of which affect your hip and then your back; some of which raise hell with your shoulders, and so on.

## The Heart Doc

Jeremy and I are out in Aspen as I write this, leading one of my Younger Next Year retreats, a five-day, "total immersion" retreat, in Aspen. This year, one of the guests is an engaging cardiologist Jeremy and I have both taken a great shine to . . . to him and his nurse-wife, actually. He is a conspicuously smart, decent guy. But here's the thing: His back and neck are a mess. Just think: He is one of the brightest, best educated (medically) guys in the country—he's a real leader in his field—and he's in this dreadful spot. He's already had two back surgeries and neither Jeremy nor I would be surprised, just looking at him, if he needed another one. How come?

Because he's busy doing his job, superbly, that's how come. And he does not think consciously about his back while he does it. There may be a bunch of causes, but one of the things he does—by the hour, day after day, for decades—is bend over some diagnostic machinery that has elements that require the doctors to wear a *heavy lead apron*. So there he is, bent intently over the diagnostic gadget, with his heavy-as-lead apron hanging from his neck, for years. And darned if his back doesn't hurt. *Huh!* Back surgeries are not going to fix that, Doc! You gotta take off your lead apron and stand up straight. Good grief! And this guy is a near-genius.

He tells us about his early problems. When he first had bad back pain (almost certainly because of the lead apron and all that), he went to a medical doctor and had an operation. The surgeon had rightly concluded that the (immediate) problem was a bulging disc. He fixed it by carving away some of the bone on the part of the vertebra that was bearing down on the disc and also draining some of the fluid from the middle of the disc to make it smaller. Problem "solved," and his back pain was much reduced—for eight years, which is surprisingly good. But it was obviously no cure and the pain reappeared, in a different disc and vertebra, and led to *a second operation*. Again, temporary relief. But Jeremy has seen him walking around, seen him doing Bill Fabrocini's warm-up exercises, and it's obvious that his back is still a mess. And it is going to stay that way until he makes fundamental changes *in his behavior*! Which, I think, he will. Jeremy and I are both fond of him, as I say, and Jeremy means to stay in touch. And the doc himself is plenty smart. Now that he's heard this "big picture" story, he gets it. "Local" fixes—including two serious surgeries—did not effect a permanent cure. Big picture *or behavioral changes are a different story*. My guess is he and Jeremy will fix it for good this time. We'll see.

So you now have a fairly sophisticated, overall picture of back pain. Now let's fix the sucker.

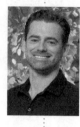

## CHAPTER SEVEN

## RULE #2

# Be Still So You Can Heal (The Neutral Spine)

**From Jeremy**

et's assume that you are beginning to get the big picture. And that you have also begun to identify the "dumb" things that you've been doing to wreck your back, *and* that you have stopped doing them. Good. Now it is time to start the healing, and that is a matter of *immobilizing your lower back or lumbar spine so it can* heal, *after all those years of doing things that hurt it.*

The analogy is not perfect, but think of your tortured back as being like a broken arm or leg. When you break an arm, say, the doc puts it in a stiff cast so you can't bang it or twist it and to give it time and rest to heal. The same with your back, except we can't do anything quite as dramatic as put you in a whole-body cast for your damaged back. What we *can* do is show you how to carry yourself so that you effectively immobilize your lower back. It's not totally easy, but it will work. And bear in mind, if you do not immobilize your back, it will not heal—simple as that. Indeed, it may get worse.

What do I mean by "immobilizing" your lumbar spine? I do not mean that you can't sit or walk or have a more or less normal life. What I do mean is that you have to be really seri-ous about *maintaining a neutral spine*, all the time. Maintaining a neutral spine is at the heart of your cure, and will be at the heart of your life after your cure. This is the time to learn how to achieve a neutral spine and how to maintain it *all the time*, even when doing various movements.

The spine is a meticulously engineered piece of machin-ery, *but* it has a lot of redundancy built in. By this I mean that unlike the knee or shoulder, in the spine when you have a bad joint, the surrounding structures can "help" bear the loads, and you can function more or less normally and without pain. Take the pressure of bad posture — and dumb movement patterns — off, and there is very likely enough "room" in this spine for the sufferer to have a normal life. For example, the "holes" where the nerves come out of the spine (the foram-ina) are *still* big enough for the nerves to exit, pain-free, if you're not squeezing the area with lousy posture. In the same vein, there is probably still enough cushion in the flattened disc to support a correctly aligned spine (but not a bent or misshapen one). And so on.

"Neutral" means the position in which the least amount of problem loads occur, all up and down the spine. The "prob-lem loads" in some pictures we've shown are extreme, but even those inflamed joints and nerve roots will likely calm down if you leave them alone for a while. Which is to say, if you keep your spine in neutral. As bad as those injuries are (and as long as it took someone to create them) there is a strong chance that that sufferer can go about his or her life, with a neutral spine, in little or no pain.

Learning to keep a neutral spine is not totally easy. And learning to maintain it all the time is harder. But this is the "cast" that lets your body heal. It is worth going to a lot of trouble to get this right. And it is a lesson that you will use for the rest of your life, long after the problem area has "healed."

Okay, step one is understanding the concept of neutral spine. Step two is learning to find it and lock it in place, and keep it in place forever (which we will teach you in Chapter 9).

The neutral spine is the position that allows your spine to do its job with the least amount of stress and load. And—if you have already damaged your back—it is the position that results in the least amount of new damage or pain.

For most people, the picture on the left is the neutral spine. The other two are not.

Note the gentle curve of the lower back in the "good" spine. For the majority of you, this is how your neutral spine will look. If you have developed significant degenerative changes or were born with significant abnormalities (it happens, but not a lot),

**Neutral Spine**

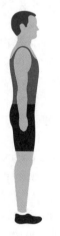 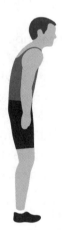 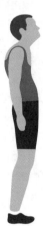

GOOD         BAD

your neutral spine may look a bit different. For now assume that your neutral spine looks like one on the guy on the left. Spines vary, and you may have your own unique neutral spine that is a little different from this. Whatever your own neutral spine, that is the position you want to maintain as you go about your daily life. It is also the position in which you feel the least pain. Again, maintaining a neutral spine is a fundamental behavioral change for most people. And it is readily doable. In a few months' time, I predict that it will be natural and you will scarcely need to think about it. One of the near-magic presences in our lives is "muscle memory." Maintain your spine correctly for a while and muscle memory takes over. *Then* it is just a question of seeing to it that your muscles are strong enough to do their job.

How do you keep your spine neutral and still be a dynamic, moving, active human being? By learning to brace your neutral spine with your core (Chapter 9) and maximizing movement in your hips (as opposed to your lower back). As Chris mentioned in Chapter 6, one of our cardinal rules is *"Thou shalt not bend or twist with thy lower back."* And you don't need to. You can rotate from side to side and bend forward and back using your hips. You do not need to flex or twist your lower back.

You may ask: Isn't range of motion important for the lumbar spine? Answer: Not really. At least, it is usually the least important factor for someone who has had significant back pain, and should be reintroduced only after pain has stopped. Most people who have experienced regular, serious back pain have already sustained significant wear and tear on the spine. The general pattern I see is a combination of two things: first, worn-down vertebral joints that are hypomobile (stiff), secondary to arthritic changes and degeneration; second, lumbar vertebral joints that are hypermobilie (loose), due to over-stretched ligaments and atrophied muscles. These problems are best resolved when we protect the spine by bracing and "locking down" the lumbar spine and moving in a manner that completely changes the axis of motion from the lumbar spine to the hips and shoulder girdle. You can eventually introduce some gentle lumbar range-of-motion exercises in non-loaded ways. This is what the "Cat/Camel" exercise that we introduce later is for. Small, gentle lumbar range-of-motion exercise is necessary for things like synovial joint lubrication, the reduction of friction between vertebral segments and discs, and disc nutrition, among other things. For example, walking requires a few degrees of freedom between the lumbar vertebral joints (3 or 4 degrees rotation) with coordinated muscle contractions to enhance stabilization and supply necessary lubrication and nutrition to discs and joints. For our purposes, we recommend keeping lumbar motion to a minimum, especially until your pain is gone. Once that occurs, you should make only healthy, non-loaded, non-repetitive lumbar movements, such as those necessary for walking and the cat and camel exercise. Spinal stability, core endurance, hip mobility, and core and gluteal strength are far more important for maintaining a healthy spine once you've had back pain. You can do just fine in life with almost no rotation or excessive movement in your lower back. Let your hips do the work, and your risk of recurring back pain is sharply reduced.

## Finding Your Neutral Spine

Finding your neutral spine can be a bit tricky for some but you can do it. Here's what you do. Lie on your back with your knees bent and your feet flat on the floor. Try to relax everything in your body, and just breathe. Then let's start by performing a *pelvic tilt*.

To do that, flatten your lower back into the floor (see top drawing), and curl your tailbone upward. This is a "posterior pelvic tilt," if you want to put a name to it. Now, arch your back so that your lower back comes off of the floor (middle drawing), and point your tailbone toward the ground (an "anterior pelvic tilt"). Now, slowly go back and forth between those two motions a few times (bottom drawing). Find the position of your lower back between these two extremes (flattening your back or arching it) that feels the most comfortable to you, and stop there. This is your neutral spine. It may take a few tries but it's not hard.

*Stop here for a second.* You have just reached an important point, and you don't want to "lose" it. Everyone's neutral spine is a bit different depending on the anatomical condition of their lumbar spine. For most people, there will be a gentle curve in

**Finding Your Neutral Spine**

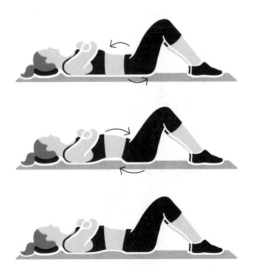

the lower back. For those who already have some kind of a disc bulge, their neutral spine might be more arched (butt more extended). For those with spinal stenosis, their neutral spine may be a little more flattened than the one in the picture on the previous page. Don't worry about it. Whatever feels the most comfortable for you is your neutral spine for now. In time, your neutral spine will likely become more like the "normal" picture as pain and inflammation subside.

Think about *your* neutral spine and assume that position all the time until it becomes second nature—until "muscle memory" takes over.

Next, we move on to a discussion of techniques to help you maintain a neutral spine. But first, Chris is going to tell you why it is very likely you haven't heard of these concepts before.

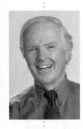

## CHAPTER EIGHT

# The Insurance Game

**From Chris**

························································································

This is an "aside" from our main thesis, but an important one. There is an "insurance game" that plays a part in the lives of almost all of us with back pain, and the game is *fixed* . . . against us. One of our goals in doing this book is to cut you loose from its tangles—because insurance today is structured to push you to do repetitive and ultimately useless fixes (not cures), and it sometimes it pushes you in the wrong (read "dangerous") direction.

Most insurers are not wonderfully straight in their dealings with certain aspects of back pain. I am not talking so much here about medical events; they are a little different. I am talking about the use of therapists and other healers, whom so many of you spend so much on.

Here is the problem. Most insurers pay for some therapeutic treatment of back pain, but the payments (like most therapies and therapists) are focused on fixes, not cures. For example, insurers pay (about $50 a treatment) for a chiropractor to do an "adjustment" of your back (i.e., he or she will "pop" your back with a high-velocity treatment of the spine or joint). A little bit of history may help here. It was once believed that when chiropractors did high-velocity treatments (i.e., "popped" your spine), they were actually straightening out a "kink." That is, you had somehow "thrown out" your back, and the chiropractor, God bless him, straightened it out again. Sounded great and, sure enough, you got some relief. Alas, that's not usually what happens, and the relief was temporary.

When chiropractors "pop" your back with the application of high-velocity manipulation (and there often is a *pop*), what they really are doing, in most cases, is restoring range of motion to a joint and/or releasing a muscle spasm. That *pop* you hear is the release of gases that build up in the joint. Restoring range of motion and releasing a spasm is a blessed relief, often enough, but it has nothing to do with curing the condition that caused the spasm in the first place. So, absent any further instructions from the therapist about behavior change, we are talking a purely palliative step.

But most insurers see additional chiropractic treatment (e.g., instruction about exercise and other behavior), which might really do some good, as just an incidental "add-on" and pay only some $10 a patient for it. For most chiropractors that won't pay the bills. Better for them to do a bunch of adjustments (or pops) and give their patients blessed relief and stay in business to help their patients another day. So even assuming that the chiropractor knows how to address serious back pain for the long haul, he or she is not really compensated to try.

The story is similarly wrong-headed but a little different with physical therapists. Therapists *are* paid to do exercise, but the payment model almost assures that they go at it in a way that is not as useful as it could be. Basically, insurers will pay for treating only *functional limitations*. That means things like being unable to sleep, turn over in bed, put on your clothes. Beyond that, you are on your own. You can't ski or jog or play with the kids? Tough . . . not covered. And your back still hurts like crazy all the time? Still no insurance. Insurance pays for only the minimum level of functionality. Therapists are not paid to analyze how you got in this jam in the first place, they are not paid to teach you how to avoid future incidents, and they are not paid to set you on a course of serious strength training of the kind that we talk about in this book, which is the only thing that is likely to effect a permanent cure, even assuming that they know how to do so.

To make things worse, many of the outcome measures mandated by insurers (to determine whether you have been returned to the minimal level of functionality) are outdated and even dangerous. In particular, the insurers often place great emphasis on *range of motion* of the lumbar spine. In Jeremy's view, this is the *least important* measure of change in most cases and may be counterproductive. The goal of sound treatment is not a more flexible lower spine; it is teaching the patient stability. So measuring recovery in terms of the flexibility of the lumbar spine is usually wrong. And urges you—and your practitioner—to try to do things you should not be doing.

Almost all medical doctors, chiropractors, and physical therapists got into the business because they wanted to help people. I hope this short chapter shows that when treating back pain, the financial deck is often stacked against them. That should change.

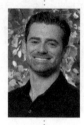

## CHAPTER NINE

# Brace Yourself

**From Jeremy**

N ow we turn to the important business of maintaining your neutral spine in a range of situations. Basically, that means *stabilizing* the neutral spine by clenching or tightening your core slightly. As if to get ready for someone to drop an orange on it. Or to tap you slightly in the gut. Over time, we want you to be able (effortlessly) to carry yourself with a slightly tightened core all the time. That's almost certainly going to take a stronger core (and one with better endurance) than what you have now. Not to worry, we'll build that, with some exercises. That, in a nutshell, is one of the most basic lessons in the book: Carry yourself all the time with a neutral spine and a slightly tightened core. And strengthen your core so that you are comfortably able to do so, all the time.

One more time: Find your neutral spine. Stabilize it with your core. Keep your core strong enough to stabilize your spine easily. Keep it up forever. Then you will be able to withstand all kind of forces, no matter how geologic. Because now you will be using your spine and your core the way they were designed to be used.

## The Body's Natural Weight Belt

We are going to be heavily focused on the muscles (and connectors) of the core, so you should have some sense of what they are. There's no need to learn the names, but we do want you to understand how they work.

Start with the ligaments. They, along with the muscles of the core, are the support beams or buttresses that hold up what would otherwise be a very whippy and flexible "tower," your spine. Without them, your spine would have the stability of, say, links of a chain. Not good. Luckily, there are many ligaments and they do a terrific job. There are not just the heavy wires that run from top to bottom. There is also an exquisitely complex and dense weave of them, right on the spine, which provide local stability.

Next come the muscles. You have layers and layers of muscles, lying crossways and other ways, to hold your spine so it's stable. (You saw these in Chapter 3. Take another look.) You know how some weight lifters wear big heavy belts when they lift? Well, you don't have to buy one of those. Nature's weight belt—the muscles of your core—will do just fine. *If* you turn them on, use them, and keep them in shape. One of my main jobs is to show you just how to do that.

*When you turn on the core muscles in the right way, it takes pressure off the discs and joints in your back and allows you to lock in your neutral spine so that you can move, exercise, and go about your day without irritating your back. With some practice, you'll be able to walk, bike, swim, lift, rotate, and climb stairs with a neutral, stable spine. Indeed, you will be able to do just about all the things you want to do, while maintaining that same neutral spine. Which means you can do them with little or no pain.*

Here is yet another critical step: learning to "engage" your core to support your neutral spine. Lie on your back with knees bent and feet flat on the floor. Find your neutral spine again, using the same technique we just talked about.

Lightly tense the muscles in your abdomen. We're trying to reach the muscles that are a layer or two down, not the ones you feel on the surface (the "six-pack"). The easiest way to tense these inner muscles correctly is to imagine that someone is about to drop an orange on your tummy. Maybe a grapefruit. Now tighten your gut, in anticipation of that odd event. *That's it.* By the way, don't go nuts by getting too tense. This should be only about 20 percent of your maximum contraction. (*That's why I said imagine an orange or grapefruit being dropped, not a bowling ball.*) To test that you're getting it right, put your hands on the inside of your hip bones, fingers pointing in and poking your belly. Now gently press inward into your abdomen. The object of this little exercise is to let you actually feel the tightening of your core.

**Engaging Your Core**

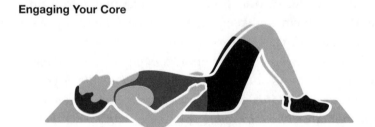

There you go. Can you maintain a normal breathing rate while you contract those muscles? If not, you are probably using your diaphragm more than your abdominal muscles. Does your stomach stick out when you try to engage those muscles? You

BRACE YOURSELF : **93**

are "bearing down" too much (think being on the toilet and straining). Try it again. Practice breathing a few times while maintaining that abdominal brace. For those who need extra help, try these visualizations. In my practice I've seen different cues help different people. Here are a few: These muscles are fairly deep down so think about trying to stop the flow of urination once you've started it. Does that help? Think if someone were going to tickle you in this position, what would you do? You wouldn't "suck in," right? You would lightly brace your abdominal muscles. That's what we are going for here. Not sure if you have it? Don't worry. We are about to do a little test to see how you're doing.

Let's challenge that neutral spine a little bit. Remember, one of the main themes of this book is to learn to *minimize movement in the lumbar spine and maximize movement from the hips and shoulders*. Keep that concept in mind as we begin this next exercise.

**CAUTIONARY NOTE**

Exercises for back pain should not make your back pain worse! You may have some aches and pains here and there as you use new muscles, but your back pain should not consistently increase as you do these. If any of these exercises makes your back worse or causes pain to radiate, stop. Either you are doing the exercises without proper form, or you are trying to perform too great a range of motion. Or maybe you're doing too many repetitions or using too much resistance. Or, face it, this just is not the right exercise for you. (It happens.) We will give you pointers throughout the book on what to do if your back is hurting with each exercise.

# Slow March with Neutral Spine

We talked about this exercise early in the book when I was describing my own back pain. You are at the point where you have discovered (or refocused on) your neutral spine and you've activated your core to support and keep the neutral spine in place. Good. Now, let's do some movements, from the hips, without moving your back.

**Step 1:** Lying on your back, find your neutral spine.

**Step 2:** Engage your core.

**Step 3:** While maintaining core engagement, slowly lift one foot off of the ground, keeping the knee bent, and without letting your lower back arch or flatten into the floor. (If your neutral spine was already flattened into the floor, that's okay; just don't push it harder into the floor when you do this.) If you can't tell whether your back is moving, put a hand under your lower back and see whether it moves when you do the leg movements.

**Step 4:** Now return that foot to the floor. Here's the hard part: Concentrate when you switch from one foot to the other not to turn off your core brace. You shouldn't feel a shift from side to side in the torso when you switch legs. Stick your hands under your lower back if you aren't sure. If you do feel lots of movement, reset and try again.

**Step 5:** Now put it all together. Try slowly "marching" with one foot and then the other without moving your lower back.

**Step 6:** Try ten repetitions.

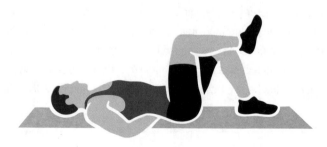

This simple exercise is *truly* worth learning and doing correctly. It is going to have a lot to do with solving your back pain.

## TROUBLESHOOTING

- Does this hurt your back? If so, stop. Relax everything. Find your neutral spine again. Does that hurt? If it does, you likely aren't in your neutral spine. Go back to the section on finding the neutral spine (page 84). If neutral spine doesn't hurt, read on.

- If you can find a position for your spine when you are lying on your back that doesn't cause pain (that's your neutral spine, of course), then chances are extremely good that you can do this march without pain. And then with a little work, chances are extremely good that you can walk, move, and go about your day without back pain! You may be able to lift your foot only an inch or two off of the ground in the beginning. That's okay! Your strength and range of motion will come as you develop more core strength and a better awareness of spinal stabilization. Stay within your pain-free range of motion.

- For some people this can take a long time. We are trying to change habits that you have been practicing for decades. It may not be accomplished in a day or week. Keep with this step until you are able to perform it pain-free. You have to build a base amount of strength sometimes before even these simple movements are possible.

# Slow March with Neutral Spine with Shoulder Movement

If you couldn't master the first movement without pain or without your back moving, don't try this one yet. For those of you who are ready, move on.

**Step 1:** Lying on your back, find your neutral spine and brace your core as before.

**Step 2:** This time, keep your legs still and just move your arms up and back from the shoulders, one at a time. This should actually be easier than moving the legs. Make sure your back isn't moving.

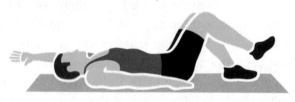

**Step 3:** Now try putting this together with the legs, moving the leg opposite of the arm you are moving, all while maintaining neutral spine.

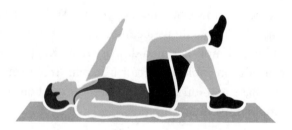

**Step 4:** Try ten repetitions.

**Step 5:** If you had pain, refer to the previous directions. Go back to legs only.

Whether or not you were able to master this exercise on the first few tries, keep reading. If you weren't able to do it, come back when you are ready to try again.

Did you finally get it? *Congratulations! You just learned spinal stability.* This is one of the key concepts in the book. You just learned to keep your lumbar spine still while moving from the hips and shoulders. If you can do that while lying on your back supported by the floor, then—with some hard work—you should be able to do that when standing on your feet and moving. Can you see the underlying concept? We are on the way. And *you* are in control.

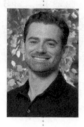

## CHAPTER TEN

# Commit to Your Core

**From Jeremy**

Y ou've learned to find your neutral spine and to lock it in. Now you are going to develop the tools you need to maintain that position and keep damaging forces away from your spine for the rest of your life. This is the all-important *endurance conditioning of your core.* As we have said, think of the core as all of the muscles between the hips and shoulders, on the front, back, and both sides. *These muscles must all act together, in sync, with equal force, to support the spine and dissipate otherwise harmful loads safely away from the spine.* Therefore, you must train all of them, not just the abs. And, you must learn to use all of them with equal force, as well. Any weak link in the chain will cause the whole system to fail and damage to the spine will occur, resulting in back pain. That means, do "whole-body" exercise.

A quick note on our goal here: We are trying to build *endurance* more than *strength. Endurance* is the ability of a muscle or group of muscles to sustain a contraction against resistance *over an extended period of time. Strength* is the ability to exert a maximal amount of force *over a short period of time.* Think for a moment about why endurance would be more important in the core muscles. How often do we need to use these muscles to sustain posture and sustain a supportive core brace? That's right—all the time. Being able to maintain a modest contraction (around 20 percent) throughout the day is far more important in the core muscles than being able to produce a maximal contraction for a few seconds.

To develop endurance, it is important to exercise the core muscles *daily.* Once you get this routine down, it will take you only about ten or fifteen minutes a day. Not a bad deal for a lifetime of back pain relief. As an added bonus, most of you will *feel better* in the morning after doing these exercises, even if you wake up with an achy back. It's a bit counterintuitive, but go ahead and do them, even if you are in pain. A strong word of advice and warning: You likely spent years performing various movements with damaging compensatory patterns. If you do these or any other exercises in this book without concentrating or thinking about it, it is very likely you will use those same compensatory patterns while performing these exercises. For example, you might use your hamstrings or back muscles when you are supposed to be using the glutes, etc. Pay close attention to the instructions and do these exercises exactly as instructed. Doing them with those faulty patterns will just make you stronger in those faulty patterns which will make your back *worse.*

The best way to develop endurance in the core muscles is with short, isometric contractions of ten to fifteen seconds. That's it. All of you type A readers pay close attention to this next sentence: Even if you can maintain a much longer contraction, only do the amount of time I suggest. Longer holds aren't better. In fact, longer holds can cause damage.

## SHORT BURSTS

**S**tudies show that maximum recruitment of muscle fibers happens in the first ten to fifteen seconds of an isometric exercise such as a plank or side plank. After that, the patient starts to fatigue and put more pressure on the discs, ligaments, and joints, which can result in irritation and inflammation. This process of muscle fatigue and joint irritation can be imperceptible to the patient during the exercise, so just take our word for it: ten to fifteen seconds, then stop. Over time, doing more can cause an increase in back pain. These short isometric "bursts" have been shown in studies to produce equal amounts of increase in endurance capacity with less damage when compared to longer holds.

Before we get to the specific exercises, let's go over some general rules:

- Always maintain your neutral spine and core brace with all exercises unless otherwise noted.

- Pay attention! Never zone out with these exercises and just try to get them over with. Think about what you are doing. Think about movement. Half the reason for doing these is to *change your behavior* regarding movement and posture. Doing these exercises every day not only builds strength and endurance but reminds you of the proper way to keep a neutral spine, brace your neutral spine, and move with the neutral spine intact.

- My suggestions for number of repetitions and amount of time are just that, *suggestions*. If you are very deconditioned (in pretty bad shape), you may need to start with less time or fewer repetitions of a given exercise. *Back exercises should never make your back hurt more.* If that happens, scale back on the number of seconds or number of repetitions. If it still hurts, go back through Chapters 7 and 9 and practice finding and maintaining a neutral spine again. If after many tries a specific exercise still hurts, then drop that specific exercise. It may not be good for your particular spine. We are not all identical.

- Know injurious pain from muscle pain. *In general,* if you feel a pain during exercise, stop the exercise. If the pain quickly dissipates (a few seconds), then it is very likely that the pain was just the pain of new muscles waking up and working. Continue on through that pain as long as it doesn't get worse. If the pain lingers for several seconds after cessation of the exercise, it could be something more serious, such as joint or nerve irritation. Stop and go back to neutral spine and try it again.

## The Seven Daily Exercises

Get used to these daily exercises, because they are going to be your friends for life. Make the commitment, here and now, to do these every day from now on. I highly recommend you do them at the beginning of your day. Don't jump right out of bed and do them, though. For various reasons, such as an increased risk of disc injury during the first minutes out of bed, you need to walk around a bit before you start. Perhaps have your coffee or breakfast first and then do the exercises before you leave the house or start your day. Is this hard? Sure, in the beginning. But after a while it becomes automatic—a pleasant and rewarding way to start your day.

**EXERCISE 1**

# Slow March with Neutral Spine with Shoulder Movement

This exercise is the one you just learned in Chapter 9 (pages 96–97). You want to remind yourself every morning about neutral spine and core bracing. Follow the steps.

Do ten to twenty repetitions—enough so that you feel you can move your arms and legs without moving your back. If you had pain, go back to legs only, Slow March with Neutral Spine (pages 94–95).

## EXERCISE 2

# The Bridge

The bridge accomplishes several things. It wakes up the gluteal muscles (the big muscles in your buttocks). It reinforces spinal stabilization. It builds endurance and strength in the muscles on the front and back of the core. And it is the precursor to doing a proper squat, which comes later in the book.

Do the bridge as follows:

**Step 1:** Lie on your back, with your arms at your side, legs hip-width apart.

**Step 2:** Find your neutral spine and brace your core to lock it in.

**Step 3:** Bend your knees and put your feet in a flexed position so that your heels are on the ground and the balls of your feet and toes are off of the ground as pictured.

**Step 4:** Squeeze your buttocks together as if you were trying to pinch a coin between them.

**Step 5:** Here's the tricky part: Using the glutes, lift your hips/torso off of the ground without moving your lower back. You should *not* articulate the spine and roll up "one vertebra at a time." You want to do the opposite of that. You want to lift the torso in one solid piece while maintaining your neutral spine. No movement should take place in the lower back.

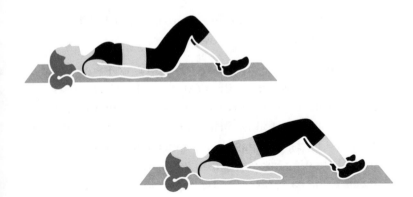

**Step 6:** Hold for five to ten seconds (remember these are suggestions. Hold to your tolerance in the beginning, with ten seconds being your goal). You should feel the muscles in both sides of your buttocks working relatively equally.

**Step 7:** Lower your back down to the starting position without losing your neutral spine. Again, do *not* articulate the spine on the way down. In other words, do not roll the spine down onto the floor one vertebra at a time.

**Step 8:** Repeat Steps 2 through 7, and do five to ten reps, with ten being your long-term goal.

## TROUBLESHOOTING

- Hamstring cramping. If your hamstrings cramp (the muscles that run down the underside of your thighs), gently push your feet into the floor away from you before you lift your hips/torso off the ground.

- Knee pain. If one or both of your knees hurt, lightly press your knees outward before lifting your hips/torso off the ground.

- Unable to maintain neutral spine. Start by trying to lift your hips/torso only an inch off the ground. Slowly progress to a full bridge over the next few weeks.

- Unable to feel glutes working. Go to Chapter 13. Then come back and start with the following regression.

- If your back hurts with this exercise, proceed to the Buttock Squeezes regression on the next page. Try these for a few days or weeks and then come back and try the bridge again, making sure to follow instructions meticulously. If your back still hurts, you may have a spinal condition like severe stenosis that makes you sensitive to extension in the spine. If this is the case, this exercise might not be for you.

### Common Mistakes

The most common mistake for back patients with the bridge exercise is that they use their hamstrings instead of their glutes to bring the hips up into position. If your hamstrings are cramping, then you aren't using your glutes enough. Go to Chapter 13 and practice "waking up your glutes," and then come back to this exercise and try it again.

## REGRESSION

### Buttock Squeezes

If you don't have the strength or control yet to perform a single bridge exercise properly for any amount of time, start with buttock squeezes.

1. Lie on your back, with arms at your side, knees bent, feet hip-width apart.

2. Find your neutral spine and brace your core to lock it in.

3. Squeeze your buttocks together as if trying to squeeze a coin between them.

4. Hold for ten seconds.

5. Do ten reps.

## PROGRESSION

### One-Leg Bridge

Once you have mastered the bridge and are able to do it with relative ease and with no discomfort in the back, you may want to progress to the one-leg bridge. You do *not* have to progress to this exercise. Depending on your spinal condition and your fitness level, you may not need to progress this far. This progression is for those who are reasonably fit and plan to be very active in sports, exercise, or outdoor activities.

1. Follow all rules for the bridge.

2. Once your hips and torso are off the ground, give extra care to make sure your core is braced as firmly as possible.

3. Slowly extend one leg at the knee without letting the hips/torso drop on that side. You will feel the glutes of the other stabilizing leg kick in as you extend the leg.

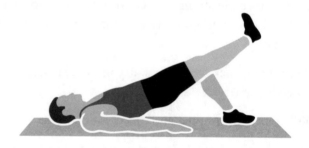

4. Hold five to ten seconds.

5. Slowly bring the extended leg back to the bent-knee starting position. (Do not lower your hips/torso while doing this. Maintain the bridge position with a neutral spine until your foot is back on the floor.)

6. Slowly lower your hips/torso back to the starting position on the floor without articulating the spine.

7. On the other side, repeat Steps 1 through 6, making sure to come up into a full bridge and lock your core in place before extending the leg at the knee.

### Common Mistakes

- When you go to one leg, it is easy to "cock" your hips to one side, to make it easier. Don't do that. Keep your thighs parallel during the whole exercise. If you can't, you aren't strong enough yet for this exercise.

- Regarding extending the leg as you come up/bending the leg down as you go down: Make sure to come up into a full bridge and lock your spine *before* you try to extend the leg. Conversely, make sure you bring the leg all the way back in before coming down to the starting position.

- Do not bring the thigh of the extended leg up. Make sure your thighs remain parallel so that you have to use the gluteal muscles to keep the pelvis stable.

## EXERCISE 3

# Crunch and Plank

We discuss these two exercises together because they both do a lot of the same things, and some of you will not get to the plank and that's okay. The plank will take you a bit further toward returning to strenuous activities, but the crunch is enough to get you out of pain. The purpose of the crunch and the plank is to build endurance and strength in the abdominal wall (crunch and plank) and glutes and lats (plank) and to increase spinal stability. Very few back pain sufferers are strong enough to do a plank properly in the beginning and must do crunches for a while before attempting the plank.

## Crunch

First of all, this exercise is not a sit-up. Sit-ups (the traditional "Army sit-up," where you pull yourself into a full sitting position) have been proven to be very risky to the spine. They run dangerous loads through the lumbar discs. If you wanted to develop a way to herniate a disc in a lab, a sit-up would be a good candidate for it. Crunches, unlike full sit-ups, do not allow movement in the lumbar spine. Your lumbar spine stays in neutral throughout.

**Step 1:** Lie on your back, with your arms at your side, legs hip-width apart.

**Step 2:** Find your neutral spine and brace your core to lock it in.

**Step 3:** Place your hands behind your head, if possible. If you can't, because of shoulder discomfort, that's okay. Find a comfortable position for your hands.

**Step 4:** Gently draw your chin in toward your neck, giving yourself a "double chin." Hold this position throughout the exercise.

**Step 5:** Slowly and carefully raise your shoulder blades and head toward the ceiling an inch or two, giving a moderate squeeze in the abdominal muscles *without flattening or rounding your lower back*. Keep a neutral spine; this will be harder than you think. Only bring your shoulders off the floor as far as you can without moving your lower back. The max distance, when you're great at it, would be no more than, say, four inches.

**Step 6:** Hold five to ten seconds, with ten being the goal.

**Step 7:** Slowly return to the starting position without moving your lower back.

**Step 8:** Repeat Steps 1 through 7, for five to ten reps, with ten being the goal.

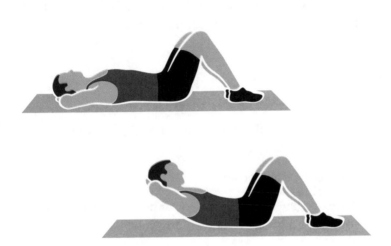

## TROUBLESHOOTING

"My neck hurts." First, you shouldn't be pulling your head with your arms. Your arms/hands are there only to provide a little support to your head and neck. Make sure that you pull your chin in toward your neck before initiating the exercise. This will engage your deep neck flexors that support the spine. If this does not relieve neck pain, move to the Regression.

### Common Mistakes

- The most common mistake is flattening or (worse) rounding the back. It is crucial that you not make this mistake. Doing crunches while continually rounding or flattening the back will promote spinal *in*stability, the opposite of our goal. Details matter!

- Chin jutting. If your chin is poking out toward the ceiling with each rep, you are not stabilizing your cervical spine and your neck extensors are taking over. Make sure to draw the chin in toward your neck before each rep.

### REGRESSION

### Abdominal Contractions

Do this exercise until you build up enough abdominal strength to accomplish the crunch.

1. Start in the same position as for the bridge.

2. Place one hand behind your lower back and one hand inside your front hipbone beside your navel.

3. Squeeze your abdominal muscles without flattening or rounding your back. You should feel your back being still with one hand and the abs engaging with the other hand.

4. Hold for five to ten seconds, with ten being the goal.

5. Repeat for several reps until fatigue sets in.

## PROGRESSION
### Plank

Once you have mastered the crunch and are able to do crunches with relative ease and without pain or movement in the lower back, try the plank. This is a great exercise to build increased core stability, endurance, and strength. Some of you (especially those with severe stenosis) may never be able to do a plank. That's okay. Give the plank a try, and if it doesn't work for you, stay with crunches. If you do go on to the plank, follow the directions closely; most people do this exercise incorrectly.

1. Lie facedown with your forehead on the floor and your arms flat on the floor on either side of you, elbows bent and palms down.

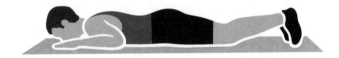

2. Find your neutral spine and engage your core to lock it in.

3. Squeeze your glutes together and squeeze your feet together.

4. Come up onto your forearms and knees with your elbows below your shoulders.

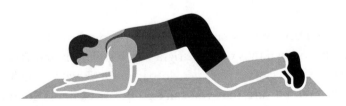

5. Lift your knees off of the floor so you are now on your toes and forearms.

6. "Traction" your forearms into the floor. In other words, press them into the floor and back toward your feet at the same time. Your forearms shouldn't move; you are just creating a pulling force into the floor and down toward your feet. This should make you feel more contraction in your lats and lower abdominal muscles.

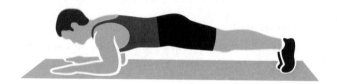

7. Hold for five to ten seconds, with ten being the goal.

8. Slowly put your knees back down first. *Do not* let your hips/pelvis go to the floor first; this would put your back into extension and may cause pain.

9. Repeat Steps 1 through 8, for two to five reps, with five being the goal.

**TROUBLESHOOTING**

- "This hurts my lower back." Some people just can't do a plank. Even if they do it the right way, it still aggravates their back. If you can't do a plank, drop it and stick with crunches. But first, be sure that you can't do it. For example, if your lower back is hurting, try sticking your buttocks in the air a little more. It could be that your hips are sagging toward the floor, putting your back into extension. Also, make sure the core is fully engaged before moving from knees to toes. Lastly, make sure you are squeezing your buttocks, which will support the lower back. If none of that works, forget it; stick with crunches.

- "This hurts my shoulders." Make sure you are tractioning your forearms down into the floor and back toward your toes. This engages the supportive muscles of the rotator cuff. If this doesn't help, try the regression that follows.

**Common Mistakes**

- Feet and legs are not together, which makes gluteal engagement more difficult.

- Back is up but the hips are dropping toward the floor. This will cause back pain in people with conditions such as stenosis or facet syndrome.

- You're forgetting to pull shoulders back and forearms into the floor with chin jutting. This will cause an increase in pressure in the shoulders and/or neck, resulting in shoulder and neck pain.

**REGRESSION**
**Plank on Knees**

If you aren't quite ready for plank but think crunch is just too easy, try this one.

1. Lie facedown with your forehead on the floor and your arms flat on the floor on either side of you, elbows bent, palms down.

2. Find your neutral spine and engage your core to lock it in.

3. Squeeze your glutes together and squeeze your feet together.

4. Come up onto your forearms and knees with your elbows below your shoulders (see second illustration, page 111, for the plank).

5. Traction your forearms into the floor, pulling them into the floor and back toward your feet at the same time. Your forearms shouldn't move; you are just creating a pulling force into the floor and back toward your feet. This should make you feel more contraction in your lats and lower abdominal muscles.

6. Hold for five to ten seconds, with ten being the goal.

**EXERCISE 4**

# Dynamic Hamstring Stretch

> ### CAUTION
>
> This exercise may irritate symptoms of people with active radiculopathy, such as severe leg/foot pain, and numbness or tingling in the legs or feet. If you have these symptoms, start with caution; you may not be able to do this exercise. If this exercise exacerbates your leg or back symptoms, skip it for now and come back to it when the symptoms are resolved.

The dynamic hamstring stretch helps to improve mobility in the hips and also helps to reinforce and strengthen your ability to maintain a neutral spine while moving the legs. It also builds endurance and strength in the core.

**Step 1:** Lie on your back and find neutral spine.

**Step 2:** Brace the core to lock in neutral spine.

**Step 3:** Bend one leg at the knee with your foot flat on floor. Straighten out the other leg onto the floor, with foot flexed (toes pointed up).

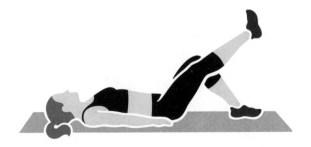

**Step 4:** Carefully raise the straight leg without losing your neutral spine; in other words, make sure your lower back isn't flattening into the floor as your leg comes up. To check, put one of your hands underneath your lower back and feel for movement. Raise the leg only as high as you can without flattening your back into the floor.

**Step 5:** Do ten to twenty repetitions on each leg. Do as many as needed to feel that you have mildly stretched your hamstrings and worked your core.

### Common Mistake

Flattening the back into the floor as you bring the leg up. Remember, one of the most important points of these exercises is to teach you neutral spine/spinal stability. You do not want to accomplish an increase of movement speed at the expense of spinal stabilization. Bring up your leg only as high as you can without flattening your back or bending your knee. Increasing hamstring flexibility will come with time.

**EXERCISE 5**

# Side Plank

The side plank works the muscles on the lateral (side) parts of the core, such as the obliques, gluteus medius, and quadratus lumborum. This exercise is a very important one. I mention this because almost everyone hates doing it. But don't give up: Your back depends on it. Many readers will not be able to do this exercise at first because their core is weak. Don't worry. There are regressions (easier exercises) for those of you who can't do this one yet.

**Step 1:** Start by lying on your side, propped up on your forearm, with your elbow under your shoulder. Relax the other arm for now. Pull your lower arm shoulder blade inward toward your spine and downward toward your buttocks, engaging the lat muscles.

**Step 2:** Drop your hips back a bit so that they sit behind your feet and shoulders.

**Step 3:** Put your top foot in front of your bottom foot.

**Step 4:** Find your neutral spine and engage your core to lock it in place.

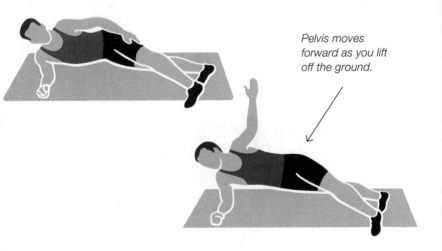

*Pelvis moves forward as you lift off the ground.*

**Step 5:** Slowly lift your hips off the ground as you bring them forward to form a straight line from foot to shoulders, like a plank. You do this to avoid side bending in the spine. This motion is the same as for the bridge except it is done on your side; in other words, you are are bringing your pelvis forward as you come up, going from bent hips to straightened hips so that you don't bend your spine sideways.

**Step 6:** If you can, raise your upper arm up toward the ceiling with the palm facing forward, and pull that shoulder blade back toward the spine and buttocks as well.

**Step 7:** Hold for five to ten seconds, with ten seconds being the goal.

**Step 8:** Slowly "sit back," pushing your hips back behind your feet and shoulders as you return to the floor in the starting position. Again, think about the movement of the bridge exercise, only done on your side.

**Step 9:** Do two to five reps on each side, with five being the goal.

## TROUBLESHOOTING

- Shoulder pain. If your shoulder hurts, make sure you pay attention to Step 1. Is your elbow directly under your shoulder? Did you pull your shoulder blade in toward the spine and down toward your back pocket before lifting up? If you feel you did these motions correctly and your shoulder still hurts, try bracing your shoulder with your upper hand as in the following picture.

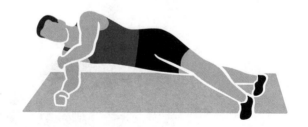

If it still hurts, move on to one of the following regressions on the next page, and perform these until you build strength in the shoulder. Then try again in a few weeks.

- Back Pain. If your lower back hurts with this exercise, try finding your neutral spine again. Try performing the exercise with a slightly more flat or rounded back and see if the pain resolves. If it does, that is your neutral spine. If the lower back pain doesn't resolve, move on to one of the following regressions, and try again after a few weeks.

- Pain on the downward side in the abdomen. This is likely muscular pain because these are the muscles you are working. Remember, if it resolves quickly once you stop the exercise, you are very likely okay doing this exercise.

**Common Mistakes**

- Starting in a "straight line" from shoulder to foot and lifting straight up from that position. This position puts potentially dangerous pressures through the spine. Instead, start with the hips back and bring them forward as you rise.

- Rolling the top shoulder forward. Throughout this exercise, make sure that your body is perpendicular to the floor and ceiling.

## REGRESSIONS

### Side Plank on Your Knees

If you are unable to perform side plank, try this one.

1. Lie on your side with your legs stacked neatly on top of each other.

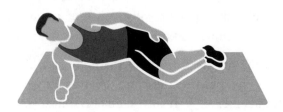

2. Bend your knees at a 45-degree angle, and drop your hips back so they are behind your feet and shoulders when viewed from above.

3. Find your neutral spine and brace your core.

4. Place your elbow under your shoulder with your forearm on the floor. Your other arm can stay relaxed in whatever position feels comfortable for now.

5. Pull your lower shoulder blade back toward your spine and down toward your back pocket and lock it in place.

6. Slowly lift your hips off the floor as you bring them forward, forming a straight line from kneecaps to shoulders, like a plank. Think of the bridge exercise, only done on your side. This is a hip movement done to avoid side-bending of the spine.

7. If you can, lift your upper arm up toward the ceiling with the palm facing forward, and pull the upper shoulder blade back and down toward the spine and buttocks as well.

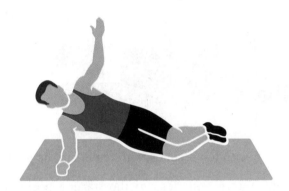

8. Hold for five to ten seconds, with ten being the goal.

9. Carefully return to the starting position by dropping your hip back while maintaining your core brace.

10. Repeat two to five times, with five being the goal.

**Modified Side Plank**

If you are unable to do the side plank on your knees, try this version, with your hip on the floor. Almost everyone should be able to do this version. Do it for a few weeks, and then go back to trying the side plank on your knees.

1. Lie on your side, supporting your head with the hand of your bottom arm (you can also use a pillow).

2. Use the hand of your top arm to brace yourself by putting it flat on the floor in front of your stomach.

3. Find your neutral spine and brace your core.

4. Slowly and carefully lift both of your thighs and legs off the floor toward the ceiling at the hip joints.

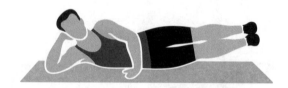

5. Hold for five to ten seconds, with ten being the goal.

6. Carefully return your legs to the starting position while maintaining core brace.

7. Repeat two to five times each side, with five being the goal.

## PROGRESSION

### Side Plank with Pull

For those of you who progress to doing the side plank with relative ease and want to pursue increased fitness and spinal stability, and are willing to accept a slight increase in risk in that pursuit, try this progression.

1. You will need a band, tubing, dumbbell, or a cable machine to perform this exercise.

2. Set the resistance to light or the weight to low to start.

3. Go into a side plank. Hold the handle of the band.

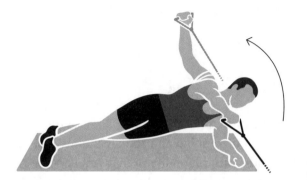

4. Without twisting the torso or moving the hips, and with your top arm straight at the elbow, pull the shoulder blade back toward your spine and down toward your buttocks. The movement occurs in the shoulder joint and between the shoulder blade and the spine. Your arm should stay straight from the shoulder down to the hand.

5. Do ten to fifteen reps on that side, then repeat on the other side.

**EXERCISE 6**

# Cat/Camel Mobilization

Okay, this is the *only* time in the book I am going to ask you to forget about neutral spine and spinal stability. This exercise is meant to build a bit of mobility in the lumbar spine and thoracic spine without loading them during the process. This is also a good way to find your neutral spine when on your hands and knees, for Exercise 7. This one is easy.

Get on your hands and knees, with your hands under your shoulders and knees under your hips. Pull both shoulder blades in toward the spine and back toward the back pockets in a "clockwise corkscrew" fashion. To get a sense of this movement, think of looking at someone's back. You would see their right shoulder blade turning in a slightly clockwise motion (left shoulder blade in counterclockwise motion) while also coming down at the same time, allowing the person's chest to stick out.

**Step 1:** Keep your neck in neutral with the rest of your spine. You should be looking down at the floor, not out in front of you.

**Step 2:** Slowly and carefully, let your stomach sink to the floor below you, creating an arch in your lower back. Go only as far as feels good.

**Step 3:** Then, slowly and carefully, push your mid/lower back up to the ceiling but only as far as feels good.

**Step 4:** Do not think of this as a stretch. Keep moving back and forth between those two positions, very slowly, getting mobility in the spine. Don't force it: This should feel good, not hurt.

**Step 5:** Notice the position that feels the best between down and up. This will be your neutral spine for the next exercise.

**Step 6:** Do ten reps. Make sure to breathe.

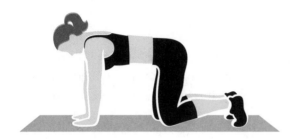

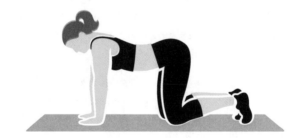

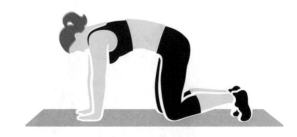

**EXERCISE 7**

# "Bird Dog," or Opposite Arm/Leg Extension

The opposite arm/leg extension exercise, otherwise known as the "bird dog," is one of the most commonly prescribed exercises for back pain. Unfortunately, it is also the one most commonly done improperly.

This exercise seeks to accomplish several things: (a) increased spinal stability when the spine is challenged from different directions with varying loads; (b) increased engagement, endurance, and strength of the back extensors including the lats; and (c) increased gluteal engagement, endurance, and strength. Done right, this exercise is a beauty.

**Step 1:** Get on your hands and knees, with your hands under your shoulders and your knees under your hips. Pull both shoulder blades in toward the spine and back toward the back pockets in a "clockwise corkscrew" fashion.

**Step 2:** Keep your neck in neutral with the rest of your spine. You should be looking down at the floor, not out in front of you.

**Step 3:** Go through the "cat" and "camel" positions to find your neutral spine.

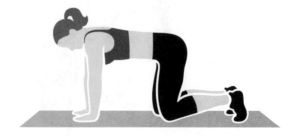

COMMIT TO YOUR CORE

**Step 4:** Lock your neutral spine in place by engaging your core.

**Step 5:** Slowly and carefully push one leg back, keeping your toes pointed toward the floor, and pushing through your heel. Make sure not to arch your back, but keep the back still in neutral spine.

**Step 6:** At the same time, slowly and carefully extend the opposite arm forward with your palm open and your thumb on top. Once your arm is fully extended, pull that shoulder blade back toward your back pocket. The muscles on top of that shoulder (upper trapezius) should not be activated. We want to activate the lats.

**Step 7:** Hold for five to ten seconds, with ten seconds being the goal. Strive for maximum engagement of the lat muscle on the extended arm and the glutes on the extended leg. Switch arms and legs without moving the back.

**Step 8:** Do ten reps on each position.

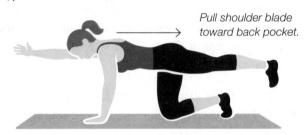

*Pull shoulder blade toward back pocket.*

## TROUBLESHOOTING

- Neck pain. You are not using your lat muscles on the extended arm and are instead using your upper trapezius muscles. This causes shoulder pain. Make sure when you get into the hands and knees position that you "corkscrew" the shoulder blades back before starting cat and camel.

- Back pain. Make sure you are in neutral spine and that the core is braced. If this doesn't help alleviate pain, go to the regressions.

- Knees hurt on the floor. Add a pillow or pad.

## Common Mistakes

.....................................

1. Internal rotation of the shoulder with palm facing down. This does not allow proper engagement of the lats. Doing the exercise this way negates some of the most beneficial aspects of the exercise.

2. Pointing toes behind you. This makes it much more difficult to engage the glutes of the extended leg. Again, this negates some of the most beneficial aspects of the exercise. Make sure toes are pointing toward the floor.

3. Arching the back during leg extension/extending the neck during shoulder flexion. If your neck or lower back is moving, this means you are not stabilizing your neutral spine. If you can't accomplish this, go to the regressions and come back to this exercise later.

4. Going through the exercise in quick reps instead of isometric holds. The exercise is meant to build endurance. Moving slowly and isometric holds are a must.

## REGRESSIONS

### Shoulder Flexion in Quadruped

If you were unable to do the "bird dog" exercise and tried the troubleshooting tips with no success, try this easier exercise and then work your way back up to bird dog in time. The goals are the same.

1. Get on your hands and knees, with your hands under your shoulders and your knees under your hips. Pull both shoulder blades in toward the spine and back toward the back pockets in a "corkscrew" fashion.

2. Keep your neck in neutral with the rest of your spine. You should be looking down at the floor, not out in front of you.

3. Go through the "cat" and "camel" positions (see Cat/Camel Mobilization, page 124) to find your neutral spine.

4. Lock your neutral spine in place by engaging your core.

5. Slowly and carefully extend your arm forward with your palm open and your thumb on top. Once your arm is fully extended, pull that shoulder blade in toward your spine and back toward your back pockets. The muscles on top of that shoulder (upper trapezius) should not be activated. We are trying to activate the lats.

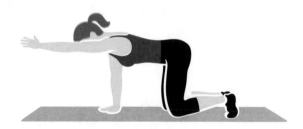

6. Hold five to ten seconds, with ten being the goal.

7. Alternate arms for ten total reps on each side.

8. Once you are able to perform this exercise regularly without pain, move on to hip extension in quadruped.

**Hip Extension in Quadruped**

This is the follow-up to the previous exercise. Once you can do this without pain or difficulty, try the full "bird dog" exercise again.

1. Get on your hands and knees, with your hands under shoulders and your knees under your hips. Pull both shoulder blades in toward your spine and down toward the back pockets in a "corkscrew" fashion.

2. Keep your neck in neutral with the rest of your spine. You should be looking down at the floor, not out in front of you.

3. Go through the "cat" and "camel" positions to find your neutral spine (see Cat/Camel Mobilization, page 124).

4. Lock your neutral spine in place by engaging your core.

5. Slowly and carefully push one leg back, keeping your toes pointed toward the ground and pushing back through your heel. Make sure not to arch your back, but keep the back still in neutral spine.

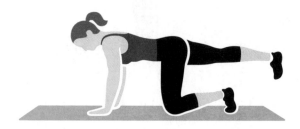

6. Hold for five to ten seconds, with ten being the goal.

7. Alternate legs for ten total reps.

8. Once you are able to complete this exercise without problems, go back and try the "bird dog" or opposite arm/leg extension (page 126).

## PROGRESSIONS

Once you are able to perform the "bird dog" with relative ease, you may want to try the following progressions to increase your spinal stability and fitness.

### Opposite Arm/Leg Extension on BOSU Ball

This exercise increases your ability to maintain spinal stability in dynamic activities and sports such as skiing, biking, or running on uneven surfaces.

1. In the gym, locate a BOSU ball. This piece of exercise equipment is that odd-looking inflated flexible half-dome that you see in most gyms. It's round on one side and flat on the other and is usually blue. Next to it, set up a step or some other surface that is one to two inches high.

2. Kneel with both knees on the BOSU ball and your hands on the step as shown in the picture.

3. Perform opposite arm/leg extensions (see page 126).

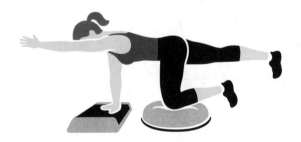

4. You will notice that with the introduction of instability with the BOSU ball, this exercise is much more challenging.

### Opposite Arm/Leg Extension with Arm/Leg Movement

This exercise teaches increased spinal stability/core control while highlighting hip and shoulder movement independent of the spine.

1. Perform opposite arm/leg extension (see page 126).

2. Once your arm and leg are extended, make sure your core is completely locked down.

3. Without moving the spine or torso, make small circles with the leg, beginning in the hip joint.

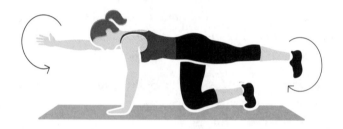

4. Do the same with the arm beginning in the shoulder joint, being careful not to move the torso.

5. Do ten circles, then switch arm/leg.

6. Alternate for ten reps.

Well, that's it for the 7 Daily Exercises. Don't be concerned if it takes you a while to get these exercises right. And don't worry if it takes a half hour or more to do them at first. Once you become familiar with them, you will be able to do them in only ten minutes each day.

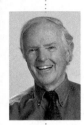

## CHAPTER ELEVEN

# Stress and Back Pain

**From Chris**

The day I sat down to edit this chapter for the last time, there was an obituary in the *New York Times* for John E. Sarno, MD, who "wrote the book" (*Healing and Back Pain*) on what he claimed (without support, I'm afraid) were the psychological origins of back pain. As the *Times* put it, he was "revered by some as a saint and dismissed by others as a quack." That is still roughly the state of his reputation today: Doctors tend to dismiss him but a lot of his patients think he's terrific. Jeremy takes a middle ground. He thinks that perhaps 10 percent of back pain has primarily emotional roots and the rest is physical. In addition, psychological elements can aggravate physical pain significantly. But 10 percent is worth a word here. More than a word, actually. Jeremy and I do not presume to give psychiatric advice—or advice about stress, which is mostly what's involved—but we include this brief chapter just to alert you to the possibility that your back pain may have its roots in stress or it may be worsened by stress or other largely psychological issues.

I confess that a couple of years ago I would have been even more skeptical than I am today about stress and, by extension, about the connection between stress and back pain. But there has been a lot of talk lately about *stress* being the great scourge of American life, especially corporate life, and the importance of "mindfulness"; there seems to be broad agreement that both are real and important. Some corporations are spending serious time trying to help their people learn mindfulness. Like others of my generation, I used to think that talk about stress (I'd never heard of mindfulness) was something made up in California by out-of-work yoga teachers, and I said the hell with it. That, it turns out, was a deeply uninformed view. Stress, I have lately learned, is very real indeed. And it probably can raise hell with your back, all by itself. Jeremy's estimate that some 10 percent of back pain is caused by stress is probably pretty good.

Stress is a fundamental part of our emotional wiring, and it runs deep. I'm going to use a little technical language here to make me sound smarter than I am. A lot of the emotional stress we face is handled by our "autonomic nervous system." How do you like that! Two branches of the autonomic nervous system have a lot to do with running emotions and related body changes. The first is the *sympathetic branch*, which basically speeds things up when life gets hairy. The other one is the *parasympathetic branch*, which basically slows things down, especially after a fight-or-flight event has made you crazy.

The parasympathetic system is for everyday use, when things are more or less okay. It handles routine stress in a routine way, and does not make you sick or crazy. The sympathetic system is supposed to be triggered only when things get seriously scary (we are talking about the sudden appearance of lions, say, or robbers with guns)—extreme situations in which it makes sense to go crazy. If there really is a lion looming in the deep grass, you've got to get *out of there ASAP*, so all the stress you can muster makes perfect sense. Same deal on the streets of the city when a thief with a knife appears out of the shadows and asks if you would be good enough to give him your wallet. Or your wife. Again, legitimate stress.

Your body does an amazing thing in those fight-or-flight situations. *Everything* is instantly rewired to give you the best shot at either fighting back or getting away. One big change is in the blood—of which there is not enough to be everywhere at once. It is shifted from peacetime distribution to a wartime footing. It is drained out of your digestive system, for example, and redirected to your extremities: legs to run for your life, or arms and shoulders and hands to grapple with the beast. And it goes to the parts of your brain and nervous system that deal with emergencies. At the same time, your heart cranks up to deliver *four or five times* as much blood to your body. The hair on your body "stands up" so it is better able to sense movement in the air (wow!). Your eyes dilate and your hearing becomes more acute. The nutrient absorption system is shut down, as are many other systems that have to do with routine maintenance. (Chronic, nonstop stress, which we'll get to in a minute, is a horror for a couple of reasons. First, you cannot be responding to those extreme conditions all the time: That would be like a muscle spasm—it starts to hurt. Second, all those routine but deeply important processes get shortchanged, and you go to hell for lack of maintenance. So . . . chronic stress is super-bad.)

When the threat passes (and if you survive), the parasympathetic system takes over and order is restored. The hair on your neck settles down, the regular allocation of blood returns, and so on. And it works like a charm for zebras and elands and such. For us, alas, not so good. As Robert M. Sapolsky tells us in *Why Zebras Don't Get Ulcers*, the zebra can be running furiously for its life one minute, and calmly cropping grass the next. Zebras are blessed with forgetfulness. Not us. We are blessed—and cursed—with the ability to contemplate and prepare for future emergencies and to hold on to and learn from past ones. We are not designed to *let go*. Eventually we do let go, but it takes us longer. So we have more stress than zebras.

We have another flaw in the way our *fight-or-flight* mechanism works. It is not just the lion or the guy with the knife that sets off our system; it's all kinds of stuff. Like competition in the workplace. Like fear of our boss. Like rejection or demotion for failure to *achieve* this or that. Which may not sound bad but it really is. Because we take that kind of stress just as seriously as we do the lion-in-the-grass type of stress. And the problem is that that kind of stress is being triggered almost constantly, in our aptly named "high stress" workplaces and society. Which leads to *chronic stress*.

Intermittent stress—the kind that is triggered when the lion jumps out at you—is useful. *Chronic stress* is a curse. Not a complete curse; it does enable "advanced" cultures like ours to focus much harder and much, much longer than humans used to do on what we want to achieve. We run our mighty engines at near-redline levels all the time and, sure enough, we tear around like crazy . . . *achieving* great things. Which is nice. And we pat ourselves on the back for doing it. (And view the French, say, with contempt because they are not as nutty as we are.) We more than pat ourselves on the back; we give each other fat salaries and tremendous recognition. Being able to function at "redline" or sympathetic nervous system levels almost all the time is richly rewarded in this country. Which is fine except for one thing: It is eating us alive. The dislocation of circulation from core to extremities, the hyper-use of the signaling system, all the profound changes that are set in motion when the lion looms short change other areas, including, interestingly enough, our lower backs. And that dislocation can cause random short circuits, muscle spasms, and weird torques to the back. And they hurt. Quite a lot. It is not the principal source of back pain, but, for those who suffer from it, it is deadly serious and is entitled to serious treatment.

How do you know if you are part of the minority for whom stress is a serious cause of back pain? Hard to say but basically it's just like what Jeremy says about back pain generally: Pay attention to the pain. Focus on the behaviors that seem to precede or go with back pain. And cut them out. If back pain is correlated with stressful situations, think about it. Maybe get yourself out of that mess. Or study one of the thousands of books about "stress management" and "mindfulness." There's a lot of material out there on mindfulness, and it is helpful.

## Stress-Induced Cardiomyopathy, Anyone?

Okay, here's my own little stress story, the one that made me seriously open to the idea of stress as a serious thing.

I was recently in the midst of a ton of heavy, work-related stuff, and we had just flown out to Aspen for a series of work meetings and such (there would be a little skiing but not much). We were starting *two* new businesses and neither was easy. Hilary and I got to the friend's house where we were staying late at night. But the real thing was that I had learned earlier that day that my beloved coauthor and friend, Harry Lodge, was going to die of cancer in the next few days. The whole business was the very definition of stress—a "perfect storm," you could say.

The morning after our late-night arrival, I was unpacking when I had a "funny feeling" in my chest. Long story short, I told

Hilary I felt weird, we called the local hospital, and soon I was on a gurney in a big ambulance being rushed to the emergency room. I was met by an absolutely terrific heart doc, a mild-mannered guy with a serious national reputation, even though he mostly practiced in a medium-size Colorado town. Lucky me. He said I was having a heart attack, and he was going to run a camera up my femoral artery (in my leg) to take some movies of my heart and put in stents to open the presumably clogged arteries . . . all the stuff I needed to, you know, stay alive.

Rats! I have always been proud as a peacock of my great heart and aerobic strength; now this! Good grief.

But it turns out it was not that bad.

"Interesting," the doc says, after I come out of the anesthesia. "You don't see this every day, but you did not have a heart attack. A heart attack is a failure of the heart, caused by a blockage of blood vessels that feed the heart. In a surprisingly short time, the part of the heart that is not getting fed—or the whole organ—dies. *That* is a heart attack and, mercifully, you did not have that. In fact, your heart and the vessels that feed it are in amazing shape: You will never have a heart attack." Oh. I took that pretty well, but I was curious, too. If I'm not having a heart attack, why are we here? "What's up?" I ask.

"Interesting," the doc says again. "I have only seen it a few times, but you have a classic case of *stress-induced cardiomyopathy . . . a temporary (and sometimes fatal) weakness of the heart itself, caused by stress.*"

"I'll be damned."

"Yes," he says, "Extremely lucky man. You have what is sometimes called 'the widow's broken heart,' common among recently bereaved spouses. Almost certainly brought on, in your case, by general stress and by concern for your gravely ill friend. [He had interviewed me briefly before the procedure.]

Sometimes it is fatal, but not for you. And, if it's not fatal, it simply goes away." I nod, but I don't begin to get it. I press for more information.

"Let's go to the videotape," he says. He wheels over this big gadget and, in a second, I am looking at a movie of my own beating heart. *Yowee!* A very rare treat. None of the many tests for heart problems goes inside and takes movies; it's too dangerous. But this was not a test, and here we are. "Here's the good news," he says, and points to what he says are the amazingly clear (unblocked) and peppy arteries all around my heart. And the strength of the muscles. Rare, he says, especially for an old chap like me. Then he drops the bomb.

"Here is *where the stress hit you*," he says, and points to the lower one-eighth of my thumping heart. "Your other heart walls are vigorous and fine, pumping lots of blood. This area, they are not. Also, you have some fibrillation, irregular beats." He points. The difference is unmistakable. For a long time we both stare at my beating heart, see the weakness and the arrhythmia. "This will go away on its own in a while," he says. And repeats how very lucky I am. Huh.

What's the point of the story? It's simple: Stress is real. You can see it in a movie of your heart. It can have a very real impact on your body. It literally weakens you and leaves you prone to all kinds of things. You can *see* stress happening on some occasions. And—maybe—there are things you can do about it. I received several serious lectures from doctors during my "widow's heart attack" phase, all urging me to remember that I was in my eighties and to, for heaven's sake, cut back some on my routine. Which I did. It's an interesting compromise between staying as alive and fully committed as possible. I'm still feeling my way. We'll see.

What about you? All we can say is, watch yourself. By which we mean, keep an eye on your own situation and bear in mind the *possibility* that your back pain *may* be stress related. Then our advice is to quit your job, get a bowl of rice, and sit on the sidewalk. Or go live with your parents. Some damn thing, I don't know. Stress is hard. But it is not imaginary. Read up on it. Do something.

Actually, we have some better advice than that. There are a lot of well-trained people—including our friend Sarah Stuart, who has done retreats and other work with me—who have studied stress and who instruct businesspeople in particular in "mindfulness," a technique that the great guru in the field, Jon Kabat Zinn, defines as "paying attention in a particular way: on purpose, in the present moment, and nonjudgmentally." Okay. But my shallow experience with it would lead me to say it is learning to do relatively short bursts when you clear your mind of all thoughts about what's coming next (or what stupid thing you did yesterday) and focusing hard on the moment. We are not going to go into any depth on this topic because I can't. But there are a ton of books out there. Do some reading.

To get an idea how pervasive a concern about stress has become, consider the fact that Division I college football players in many schools devote twelve minutes a day to practicing meditation for stress relief, and they say it helps a lot. Meditation is all over the place. We gently submit that it is well worth it to almost all of us to take a look at stress in our lives. And for those of us with serious back pain, we should try to figure out if we are part of the small minority whose back pain is primarily emotionally based.

One more bit of isolated information. The great goal in stress management is to enhance your *resilience*: your ability to switch quickly from the sympathetic to the parasympathetic nervous system. And that lovely gift turns out to be *trainable*. I am sure you will be thrilled to learn that what you are doing is training your "vagus nerve" (a nerve in your brain that regulates this stuff). A "higher vagal tone" means you have "greater calm and resilience," and so on. Again, I'm in no position to prescribe here, but I urge you to look at some of the many books on the subject. I will note that they often recommend a lot of slow breathing, which I used to think was stupid. Wrong again. It is apparently the case that doing breathing exercises—and especially going slow on the exhale—actually heightens your vagal tone. *So does exercise.* A few years ago, a heart doc said that I had "a high vagal tone, common amongst serious athletes." Not quite high enough, apparently, to see me through this recent crisis.

Does all this stuff matter? Well, yeah. I have read that, by one measure, one person may be *thirty times as resilient* as another. Of course, my pathetic competitive juices started flowing: I wanted to be more resilient. I thought maybe it would not be so bad to be, say, *thirty times as resilient* as the other kids. Super-important for serious executives, hotsy-totsy litigators, and, maybe, you and me.

Listen—big caveat: This is anything but a comprehensive and well-informed discussion. What I do hope is that there has been enough here to catch your interest and get some of you to dig further. Stress is very real indeed, dealing with it is trainable, and some level of stress-avoidance and mindfulness will help.

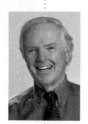

CHAPTER TWELVE

# Develop a Habit: Do It Forever, or You're Cooked

**From Chris**

Our great worry with this book—Jeremy's and mine—is not that the exercises and so on won't work; they will. It's *you* we worry about. Will you take us at our word that the *only* way to cure back pain forever is to do it yourself ... to change your own behavior and to do the damned exercises? Maybe, maybe not. We worry that you just won't get it. Or have the resolve and, well, *character* to act on it. In this country we are so used to having doctors and other healers do it for us that it is hard to get our arms around this notion. And—as a society—we are a bit idle. We work like crazy at our jobs (maybe too crazy) but not on our bodies or ourselves. Well, if you are going to heal your back pain, you're going to have to change that.

The fact is—and we have not come right out and said this before—it makes awfully good sense to do these exercises six days a week. For the rest of your life. That is familiar advice to me. It is exactly what we recommend for the general population in the Younger Next Year books and especially in the excellent *Younger Next Year: The Exercise Book*, all of which we recommend warmly. But if this is new dogma to you, I would not be stunned to learn that some of you are choking, ever so slightly, on the concept. "Six days a week?" you say to yourself. "Forever, huh?" "Stern," you mutter to yourself; "very, very stern." And you do what you've done a thousand times before: You make a *tiny, private adjustment*—somewhere in the back of your mind, where cowardice and self-preservation meet—a private adjustment that says, "That *has to be* nonsense at some level, a first offer in a negotiation that *has* to get more sane than *that*! Here's what I will do: I will simply do the best I can. Then we'll see. And don't forget: Something is always better than nothing."

Perfectly sensible. I don't blame you for one second. All of us make little accommodations with perfection all the time, to keep from blowing our brains out or lapsing into terminal self-hatred. Fine. I have made thousands of such deals myself, maybe a million. And I strongly suspect that they have kept me alive and happy.

*But not this trip. Failure to honor* this one *is going to make a hash of your life.* Jeremy's injunction is *not* an opening position; it is *the way, the truth, and the light.* It really, really is. Ignore this one and you will get messed up fast. You will tumble back into pain in no time and have to start all over again. In agony. And that first sweet flush of recognition and resolution that you got from reading this book will be lost forever. It is like weight loss. If you make a new resolution to lose weight every single morning, you will never, never do it. The first time is not necessarily the last, but it is as easy as it is ever going to get. So, my strong advice on this one is: *Make a decision now. Hang on to it like grim death. And never, never let go.* It may get more important down the road, as your body goes to hell, but it will never get easier. *Now is the time,* honest. *Don't be a dope.* Do these exercises every day for the rest of your life. You want *permanent back pain relief? Study the book and do these exercises forever.*

## Six Things to Think About

Jeremy is, of course, the expert on all things substantive. But I am a bit of an expert on making excuses to yourself, falling off the wagon, and, you know, generally going to hell. And, oddly, I am also a bit of an expert on how *not* to do all that. Here is what you need. You need to *believe*, and I suspect you are pretty far down that road. Then you need to have *structure*. We'll talk about that. And you need to have a deeply engrained *habit*. Here are six things to think about while you are trying to do all that.

First, a touch of good news. Developing a serious exercise habit is one of the *easiest* of all those things you ought to be doing but are not. Getting a don't-eat-garbage habit (or dieting) is inexplicably hard and most people fail at it. Giving up the second or third glass of wine? Same thing. But exercise is comparatively easy. Not sure why but one reason is it is *doing something*, and that is so much easier than promising *not to do* something . . . denying yourself. Sounds silly but you can just plain make up your mind and *do it*. Like the Nike slogan: *Just Do It!*

Second, there's this: A good exercise habit *feels good*. Hard to believe now, maybe, but—once you get so you can do this easily—it is kind of fun. No way to persuade you about that now, except to say "Trust me, it's true. Been there and I know."

Third, it's only ten minutes a day, for heaven's sake. It will take longer when you're learning how, but after you get the hang of it, that's all it will take. Hell, you can hold your breath for ten minutes a day. No, you can't, but you know what I mean: Ten minutes ain't long.

Fourth, it is important to stress that the exercises themselves *are not that hard*. In the beginning, if you are in pathetic shape, they may be hard. Jeremy tells me that a lot of you simply are not going to be able to do them, as prescribed, for a while. And let's be realistic: That is apt to be depressing . . . it will feel like a little failure, every morning. Well, tough. You *will* get there in a couple of weeks or a month, and you know that every day that you *try*, your feet are on a sacred path: a path away from agonizing back pain and toward a decent life.

Here's a bit of strictly personal encouragement. I am not the most disciplined guy you ever met. I was never an athlete, and now I am roughly 117 years old. Okay, eighty-three. And *I* can do them. Do 'em with ease, to tell the truth. So, believe me, you can, too. And once you get there, it is not painful or even unpleasant. In fact—let me repeat this because it is so important—they feel good. It feels good to feel your core tightening beneath you. It feels good to *use* those mysterious muscles, like your glutes, which are so central to the good life. There is going to be a little surge of pride, most mornings, as you go about it . . . get it right . . . do your body and yourself this enormous favor, with so little effort.

Fifth, the exercises lend themselves to structure. You mostly don't have to *go* someplace (the gym) to do them. You don't have to struggle to fit them in when you're traveling. You can set a time and place for them and never have to *decide* again. You don't want to have to make a fresh decision about stuff like this every day. Make it automatic, like brushing your teeth. My recommendation: Make it a standard part of your early morning ritual. What I do—and what I bet will work for you—is get up, make coffee, and drink it. Cast an eye over the paper but don't read it. Personally, I don't eat breakfast. (And *please* don't kid yourself that you need food for strength, or even water for hydration first; that's simply not true.) Do the damned old exercises and get 'em over with. *Then* have breakfast, read the paper, walk the dog, or whatever you have to do.

Sixth and last, make this "*your job!*" As we've said in the original *Younger Next Year* book, one of the things that most of you (the kind of people who get into our books) have going for you is a *work ethic*. Some people do not know about that. You do; it's as natural for you as breathing. You get up every day and go to work. Probably on time. If you have that going for you, it is an inestimable advantage. You do not have to make up your mind to go to work every day, for heaven's sake; you just *do it. Use that work ethic edge.* Make these exercises *part of your job.* And do them every morning as automatically, as mindlessly, as you get up every morning and go to work. That'll see you through.

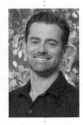

## CHAPTER THIRTEEN

# Use the Power in Your Posterior

**From Jeremy**

Possibly the most overlooked bit of anatomy, for back pain, is your backside. We are talking about your butt and especially your glutes, the big muscles that constitute most of your butt. The difficulty is that, in modern times, we have mostly used our glutes to sit on. They have atrophied as a result. The use of the buttocks exclusively as a seat cushion is a recent development in evolutionary terms, and a rotten one. It is handy, lord knows, but that wasn't the original design idea, and we are paying a horrendous price for it, mostly in back pain.

Letting your glutes go to hell in idleness ("gluteal amnesia," as the great student of back pain Dr. Stuart McGill called it) is an absolutely dreadful idea. By all means, continue to sit on them. But do much, much more, too. Remember that the glutes are the biggest muscles in your body, they have serious loads to bear, and it is critical that we let them do it. Because, if we don't, our spines (and the tiny muscles around them) will carry those loads, and they are *not* designed for it. They protest . . . they hurt. And they will continue to hurt until you wake up your glutes and let them do their job.

The gluteal muscles are a group of three muscles that make up the buttocks. There are several smaller muscles back there as well, including the piriformis. They look like this (see diagram below).

In a healthy person, the gluteal muscles perform a bunch of important functions. Here's what they should be doing:

- helping you to stand up and maintain erect posture
- keeping you from falling forward when you walk or run
- keeping your pelvis from collapsing when you are standing on one leg or walking when only one foot is in contact with the ground
- helping you to rise from a seated position
- helping you pick things up
- helping you climb stairs, ski, run, row—and that old favorite, make love

**Gluteal Muscles**

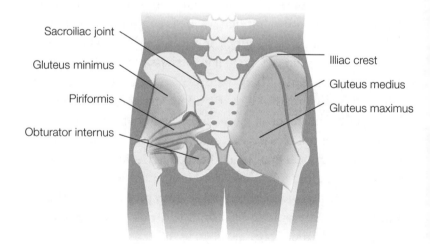

Sacroiliac joint

Gluteus minimus

Piriformis

Obturator internus

Illiac crest

Gluteus medius

Gluteus maximus

All kinds of things. Obviously, these are some of the most important things you do and these are some of the most important muscles in your body.

When you let your glutes go to sleep, things get bad. They "forget" all those critical functions, and the muscles that take up the slack are not up to the job. As we compress the muscles (by sitting on them), nerves and blood vessels in the gluteal muscle don't work as well. Our brain literally loses its connectivity with them. The muscles, and the neural pathways, atrophy (or "lose preference"); the brain "forgets" them. Hence, the term *gluteal amnesia*. In my experience, there is a very high correlation between the glutes going to sleep and back pain. *Very* high.

Here's why: When those big powerful muscles aren't doing their job, the spine takes over. It bears the brunt of the forces that the glutes are supposed to be handling and it gets overwhelmed and damaged. Instead of using those big muscles to do things like pick up your child or grandchild, you *first* use the tiny muscles around your spine to do them, and those muscles can't handle it. They become strained (which causes pain, all by itself) and eventually fail. Then things get quite a bit worse. When those little muscles fail, the forces that your glutes were supposed to be handling get transmitted directly onto your discs, joints, ligaments, and tendons. That is not what they are supposed to do and it causes serious problems. Conversely, those big psoas muscles get reflexively tighter, putting more pressure on the spine. Think about it: Every time you get out of a chair, pick something up, tie your shoe, or climb the stairs, you are putting a ton of pressure on your spine *that it is not designed to bear*. You can do it for a while. You can do almost *anything* for a while. But over the days, months, and years, these micro irritations add up to *macro* damage. Remember Chris's explanation of "geologic time"? Mountains are ground down to rubble in geologic time. Your spine is ground down to rubble in your own version of geologic time, if your glutes don't do their job.

Summary: Letting your glutes go to sleep is a terrible idea. Reversing that process and waking them up is crucial to healing back pain. Once those muscles wake up and start doing their intended work, the muscles that do the opposite motion on the joint, the psoas muscles, reflexively loosen up. If you didn't know this, don't feel bad. A lot of therapists and doctors don't know it, either. Or don't treat it effectively. Teaching you how to treat the problem effectively is one of the most important things we do in this book.

Here's what you need to do, in three steps: *Wake up your glutes, make them strong*, and *learn to use them at the appropriate times, as they were designed to be used*.

## PART ONE: WAKING UP THE SLEEPING GIANTS

You tried using your glutes with the bridge exercise (page 103). Now let's try a different way to wake them up. If you had trouble with the bridge, don't worry. We will come back to that shortly.

## Clamshell

Now, on to the all-important "clamshell" exercise. It is critical— boring and often poorly performed, *but* it wakes up *and* strengthens your glutes.

**Step 1:** Lie on your side with your hips and knees bent as shown.

**Step 2:** Take the thumb of your top hand and dig it inside your upper hip bone, as in the drawing.

**Step 3:** Lay the four fingers of that hand across the outside of your hip, as in the picture.

**Step 4:** For most of you, your middle finger (or first or third) will be lying right on the gluteal muscles we are trying to wake up. Poke your fingers in there and feel them. Reestablish that connection with your brain. Keep your fingers there.

**Step 5:** Find your neutral spine and brace your core.

**Step 6:** Slowly and carefully raise the knee, opening up your legs like a clamshell. The knee should not come toward the body but slightly away, as in the drawing.

**Step 7:** Repeat this movement for ten to twelve repetitions. Do you feel the muscles under your fingers working? If not, repeat Steps 1 through 6, or go to Troubleshooting, on the next page. Once you get it, try a few sets on each side until you feel a good burn in those muscles.

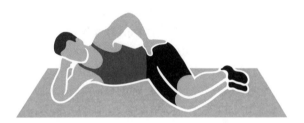

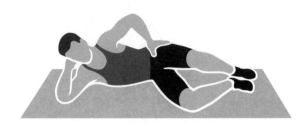

## TROUBLESHOOTING

- "I feel it down my leg or into my knee instead of in the glutes where my hand is." It is likely that you are bringing your knee up toward your torso instead of out and away from your body. Have a friend or loved one watch you do the exercise and pay close attention to the angle of movement. If you still can't get it, you may have what are called "trigger points" in the gluteal muscles. (See the next chapter, titled "Trigger Points: Muscle Pain and Back Pain" and then come back and try this again.)

- "I don't feel anything happening back there or anywhere." This is common. If you don't feel anything anywhere, keep working at it a few days. Eventually, you are likely to start to feel those glutes working. If you don't after a few days, see the next chapter on trigger points and come back.

All right, back to the bridge exercises, which you should do right after doing the clamshells (see the bridge, page 103). You should really be able to feel the glutes now when you squeeze them together before lifting your hips/torso off of the floor.

The more you practice this, the more you should feel them and the less you should experience hamstring cramping. Also remember the little trick in Chapter 10 (Bridge, under Troubleshooting) about pushing out and away from yourself into the floor to relieve hamstring cramping.

Now that we have awakened those atrophied glutes, let's move on to Part Two: strengthening them.

## PART TWO: STRENGTHENING THE GLUTES

The following exercises build strength in the glutes. An important point here is that, unlike with the Seven Daily Exercises, we are now trying to build strength instead of endurance. Therefore, you aren't going to do these every day. You need a day or two for recovery with these. I recommend doing these three times a week on nonconsecutive days. If you are worried about keeping all of this straight, don't. We have summarized your routine for you in the Appendix.

# Clamshell with Resistance

You have two options here. You can either start by holding a two- to five-pound dumbbell (depending on your strength) on your knee as you lift (see picture). Or you can buy a band to put just above the knees. Most gyms have bands, and you can buy them all over. Note that resistance of the bands varies according to color. Start with the lightest resistance and work your way up.

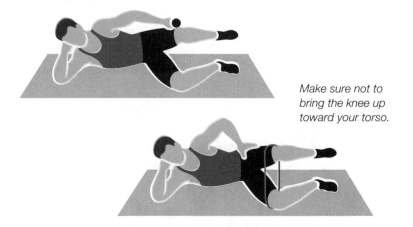

*Make sure not to bring the knee up toward your torso.*

**Step 1:** Go through the directions for clamshell (page 150).

**Step 2:** Before starting the exercise, either put the dumbbell on the bend of your top knee or place the band around your legs just above the knees.

**Step 3:** It is likely this will be harder than you expect, even with a very light dumbbell or light resistance band. *Make sure* not to sacrifice proper form just to get in a few extra reps. If you can't do the exercise properly with resistance, then you aren't ready for it yet. Either lower the resistance or go back to no resistance until you can do it perfectly. Again, try to do these every other day or so (about three times per week) for now.

**Step 4:** Do ten to twelve repetitions for two to three sets on each side, with three sets of twelve reps the goal.

## Quadruped Hip Extension

This exercise strengthens the gluteus maximus (the biggest of the gluteal muscles) as well as other muscles. Many back pain sufferers find this exercise difficult, so make sure you feel the glutes working during the clamshell exercise before attempting this one.

**Step 1:** Get on your hands and knees as you did with "bird dog."

**Step 2:** Find your neutral spine and brace your core to lock it in place.

**Step 3:** Keeping the knee bent, push your heel up toward the ceiling *without arching your back.*

**Step 4:** You should feel the contraction in the buttock far more than in the hamstring or the back.

*Do not arch back.*

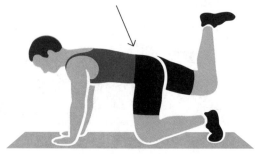

**Step 5:** Come back to the starting position without losing your neutral spine. Do ten to twelve repetitions.

**Step 6:** Switch sides and repeat Steps 1 through 5.

**Step 7:** Do two to three sets on each side, with three being the goal.

## TROUBLESHOOTING

- "My hamstrings are cramping, or I feel it only in my hamstrings." This is very common. This may take a lot of practice for you. Try lessening the range of motion, only slightly bringing the knee off the floor. Concentrate on the glute. If you can support yourself on one arm in this position, poke yourself in the buttock while making the movement to try to "wake up" the glutes. If you cannot support yourself on one arm in this position, try the standing regression below. If that does not work, go through the trigger point chapter (Chapter 14) and then return here and try again.

- "My low back hurts." This one is easy to fix. You aren't maintaining neutral spine and you are arching your back. Perfect neutral spine on your back while marching in place (Chapter 9) and then try this again.

## REGRESSION

### Standing Hip Extension

For those of you who couldn't do the hip extension on your knees for whatever reason, try this. Performing this exercise will teach you to feel the glutes working. Just like the others, it is possible to do this wrong, so make sure you pay close attention.

1. Find a chair or near-waist-height stable surface to aid in balance.

2. Find neutral spine and brace your core to lock it in.

3. With one hand, place your thumb on the bone on the side of your hip and lay your fingers across the buttock. Apply pressure with the fingers into the muscle of the buttock.

4. Slowly and carefully extend your leg backward, pushing through the heel. Feel the glutes engage beneath your fingers while the leg moves backward. This is what we are going for in the quadruped hip extension.

5. Do ten to twelve repetitions. Do two to three sets, with three being the goal. Focus on activation of the gluteal muscles.

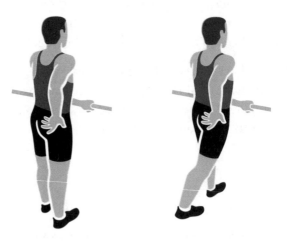

6. Once this exercise becomes easy and you feel the glutes working, go back and try the quadruped hip extension (page 154).

7. If you are unable to feel the glutes working after several tries, read the trigger point chapter (Chapter 14), and then come back and try again.

. . . . . . . . . . . . . . . . . . . . . . . . . . . . . . . . . . . . . . . . . . . . . . . . . . . . . . . . . . . . . . . .

**PART THREE: LEARNING TO USE THE GLUTES**
The goal of all of these exercises is to learn to use the glutes at the appropriate times and to build the strength in them to be able to do what's needed. This next bit teaches you the real day-to-day stuff that is so important. After you've built up some strength in those glutes, it's time to put them to use.

. . . . . . . . . . . . . . . . . . . . . . . . . . . . . . . . . . . . . . . . . . . . . . . . . . . . . . . . . . . . . . . .

## Squatting

*Pay attention! This is the granddaddy of all movements for which you need to use the glutes.* Think about the number of times you do some sort of squat in a given day. Getting off the couch, getting off the toilet, getting out of the car; picking up something off the floor. And *skiing*. On and on. *Squatting*: Done the wrong way, squatting will cause countless micro aggravations to your back and knees. In geologic time, these can be a major contributor to your hurting back. Done the right way, squatting builds the gluteal muscles and takes the load *off* the spine and knees.

To do squats correctly, it's easiest to break them down piece by piece. First (carefully and only if you are comfortable with it), do a few squats without any instruction from me. Do ten or twelve of them. What muscle group did you feel working the most? Most of you are going to say the quads (the big muscles on the front of your thighs). Some of you might say the hamstrings, some the knees. Those are all typical responses, which, alas, means you aren't doing them the proper way. If you said the glutes, you're a step ahead of everyone.

If you are doing a squat the right way, you should feel the glutes working more than the quads, say 60/40 or 70/30. Think of this as a *squat back*, not a *squat down*. In other words, you are sticking your buttocks out behind you, not down below you. Let's break this down into steps. Practice each step several times until you get it.

STANCE:

1. Stand with your feet shoulder-width apart. This means you should be able to draw an imaginary line straight down from the outside of your shoulder to your outer heels.

2. Find your neutral spine and engage your core to lock it in place.

3. Bend your knees very slightly.

4. Your feet should be pointed mostly forward. Slightly out-turned is okay but only a few degrees. Outwardly turned feet (think ballerinas) make gluteal engagement difficult. Just because something is good for a sport or activity like ballet doesn't mean it's good for your body. It's the same with golf: The best golf swing is the worst for your back.

**Step 1**

1. Stick your buttocks back behind you while maintaining a neutral spine as if you were aiming for a chair to sit down on.

2. At the same time, straighten your arms out in front of you, thumbs pointing up, as a counterbalance.

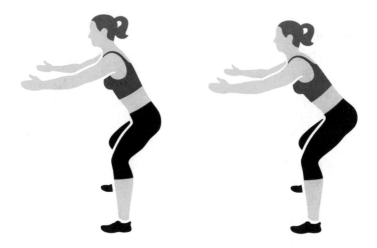

3. Don't squat down at all. Just stick your buttocks back without moving your low back.

4. This is called a hip hinge. The axis of movement is at the hips, not in the back.

5. Practice this several times until you can do it without pain and without moving your back.

### Step 2

1. Now add just a little bit of squat to it.

2. Bend the knees a little more, which will take your buttocks farther behind you and your body lower to the floor.

3. Your knees *should not* come forward—not at all is best but a little is okay. Your lower legs should be perpendicular to the floor.

4. Go only as low as you can without your knees coming forward. If your back or knees hurt a little bit, hang in there until we get through this. Step 3 will likely take away the knee and back pain.

5. Practice going up and down a few times, making sure to stick your buttocks back behind you as if you were going to sit in a chair behind you. It's okay to start with a very small range of motion.

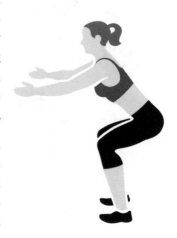

### Step 3

1. Here's the crucial and difficult part: activating the glutes as you rise from the squat position.

2. Squat down as you did in Step 2. Pause at the bottom of the range of motion.

3. As you start to rise up, push outward on the knees/heels while you bring the hips forward as if you were trying to "spread the floor" apart. Another good cue is this: Picture a piece of paper on

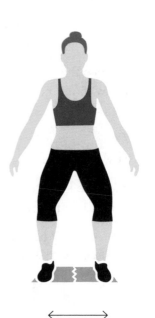

the floor on which each of your feet are on the outside edge. As you rise up and bring your hips forward, you want to rip the paper apart with your feet (your feet don't actually move; you are just pushing outward on them into the floor).

4. At the same time, you are pressing outward/spreading the floor/ripping the paper in half. Squeeze your buttocks just like you do in the bridge exercise. Use the gluteal muscles to bring your hips up and forward to the starting position. Try this several times.

5. Can you feel the glutes engaging? This is tricky. You should now feel the glutes working more than the quads. If not, read through this exercise again and try it a few more times. If you can't get it, go to Troubleshooting, following.

6. If your back or knees hurt before, does engaging the glutes get rid of or significantly decrease the pain? It should. If not, try this exercise a few more times. If it still doesn't, go to Troubleshooting, following.

## TROUBLESHOOTING

- "I'm not feeling the glutes engaging." This issue is common and it may take time to master this exercise. You are trying to change a good many years of behavior here and it isn't going to happen overnight. Try these first:

  - Make sure the feet are turned forward, not outward.

  - Make sure your knees aren't coming forward over your toes as you squat back.

- Make sure you are lightly pressing outward on your knees and/or heels (try both: some cues work for some people and some don't) as you bring your hips up and forward.

- If you still can't feel them, go back and try a few clamshells, bridges, and hip extensions, and then come back and try again.

- If it still doesn't work, go to the trigger point chapter (Chapter 14) and then try again.

- "My knees and/or low back hurt." Keep in mind that a very small percentage of people may never be able to squat pain-free. That being said, the vast majority of you will be able to squat to some degree with little to no knee or back pain. Pain in the low back usually means you aren't maintaining neutral spine and/or you aren't engaging the glutes, which is putting too much load through the spine. See the first troubleshooting item and make sure you are engaging the glutes. Try squatting with a very small range of motion for a time, slowly increasing your range of motion over the coming weeks. If your knees or low back still hurt, go on to the trigger point chapter (Chapter 14) and then come back and try this again.

# Split Squat

The last "glute integrated" movement we will cover in this chapter is the split squat. There is an "added plus" to learning this one: For many back pain sufferers, the split squat offers a painless way to get up off of the floor. We'll go over applied movement in a moment, but first try this (admittedly challenging) exercise.

Many of you have probably heard of the "lunge" exercise. The split squat is the precursor to the lunge. If you know what a lunge is, think of the split squat as a lunge in which your feet stay in place. The key (and the challenge) is to use the glutes (in the rear leg), not the quads (in front) to bring your body up.

**Step 1:** Stand with feet shoulder-width apart.

**Step 2:** Find your neutral spine and engage your core to lock it in place.

**Step 3:** Step forward, putting one leg in front of the other, about two feet apart, depending on your height. The distance between your feet is likely going to be slightly greater than you naturally want. Step out of your comfort zone a little bit. If you are worried about falling you can hold on to something to help you balance. Try to distribute your weight evenly on both feet. This is your starting position for the exercise.

**Step 4:** Slowly and carefully lower your torso toward the ground. Don't bend forward, just lower straight

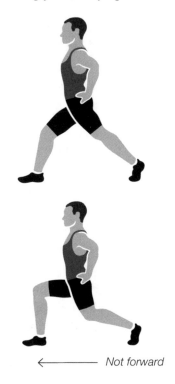

← ———— Not forward

down. Think of an elevator. If you can, go down so that the top half of your front leg (your thigh) is parallel with the floor and the lower part of your front leg is perpendicular to the floor.

**Step 5:** As you are going down, bend your back knee so that it points straight toward the floor (not forward).

**Step 6:** Here's the hard part: As you start to rise, initiate the movement with the *glutes of your rear leg*, not the quads (thigh) of your front leg.

Read that again: It's counterintuitive. Use the glutes of the rear leg to pull yourself, relying as little as possible on the quads. Aim for a 60/40 ratio (or even a 70/30 ratio) of glutes to quads.

**Step 7:** Come up to the starting position, maintaining a neutral spine and engaged core. Your feet should never move out of starting position.

**Step 8:** Repeat for ten to twelve reps, and two to three sets, with three being the goal.

## TROUBLESHOOTING

- "I don't have the balance." In the beginning, hold on to a table, chair, etc., until you develop the engagement and strength of the glutes. Your stability/balance will improve as you learn to use these muscles.

- "My knee(s) hurt(s)." Guess why? I'm starting to sound like a broken record here. Your glutes aren't working. Take one hand and press into the glutes of the rear leg as you do the exercise. Do you feel them tightening? Your hip should be extending as you come up. If you don't feel the glutes tightening as you rise, go back to the standing hip extension (page 155) for a while, and then try this exercise again after you feel the glutes working in that exercise.

You may have struggled with this chapter. That makes sense: Your glutes have atrophied and these are glute exercises, so of course they're hard. Your glutes atrophied because of years and years (geologic time for you) of poor spine habits and behavior.

You are not going to correct this in a day or a week. Keep working at it. Eventually, your glutes *will* "wake up," you *will* be able to do these exercises and movements, and your back (and your life) will be much better. Combined with the daily *core* exercises, these are the foundations for your recovery, if you have a glute problem. You have to do the exercises in Chapter 10 (core) and this one religiously. Read the rest of the book but make these chapters the heart of your routine.

If you did struggle with this chapter, the next chapter may help. "Trigger points," spasms or "knots" in the muscles of your butt, can be a significant barrier to waking up and using the glutes. Read about them and see if that's part of your problem. Then come back and try this chapter again.

## CHAPTER FOURTEEN

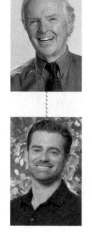

# Trigger Points: Muscle Pain and Back Pain

........................................................................

**From Chris and Jeremy**

M ost of us—the newcomers anyway—tend to think of back pain as something that is largely in the spine itself. The bones, discs, ligaments, and nerves. But what most of us don't focus on are the surrounding and supporting muscles. Which is a mistake, because they can be a major source of back pain (or something that can *pass* as back pain). And getting "right" with those muscles can be mighty important.

To be accurate, back pain is almost always a not-so-pleasing blend of muscle pain, joint pain, nerve pain, and other pain. This can be a little confusing. All pain is *transmitted* by nerves. When we speak of muscle pain or nerve pain, we are referring to the primary source of pain—that is, the pain-generating tissue. Sometimes an aggravated nerve is the source of pain so it is referred to as nerve pain. In this chapter, we are talking about pain whose primary source is muscles. Even though the pain is transmitted to your brain via nerves, the tissue that's causing the pain is muscle tissue, so we refer to it as muscle pain. It is helpful to think of that which is *primarily* muscle pain differently, because it manifests itself differently, and Jeremy's approach to it is different, too.

There's good news and bad news here (wouldn't you know it). The bad news is that muscle pain is harder to locate and trickier to fix in the first instance. The good news is that it is actually *easier* to fix in the long run, and your prospects of a *complete* cure are much better.

Which is not to say it does not hurt like blazes. Up in the 8–10 range, on a scale of 10. But often the relief can be sudden and nearly complete. You still have to do serious stuff to keep it from coming back once the fix is made, but that's always true.

## Muscle Pain

People in the healing professions refer to muscle pain both as "myofascial pain" and "trigger point pain." For laymen like you and me, "trigger point pain" may be the more useful name, because it feels like that—something that gets "triggered" by some silly move you made. Whatever we call it, trigger point pain has been a somewhat controversial topic for decades, mostly because no medical discipline claims ownership of the muscular system. Doctors are far more concerned with the joints, bursae, ligaments, and nerves. There has not been as much study of the muscular system and trigger point pain. But there has been enough, so that there is broad agreement on many points. And the best practitioners, and Jeremy in particular, have seen a lot of it.

So, what is it? Here's Jeremy: "Trigger points are tight, painful bands of muscle tissue that have predictable and recognizable patterns of pain." To put it another way, they are muscle spasms (not quite right but close enough), which is what you get when a muscle or muscle segment seizes up, under pressure, and won't let go. It's like those cramps you sometimes get in your leg, except it doesn't go away and the pain can be horrendous. Unbearable, some of the time. These spasms or cramps not only cause terrible pain in their own right, but they can change the way some joints function. As Jeremy puts it, "They also limit range of motion and change the normal distribution of loads on nearby joints, which can also cause pain." So trigger point pain is serious, and it has more than one way to grab you. If it has started to affect the range of motion of the nearby joint, in the way Jeremy suggests, clearing it up is harder, but the approach is the same.

One thing to bear in mind is that trigger points basically "lie" to us. That is to say, the obvious pain may crop up away from the actual trigger point itself. For example, the trigger point may be in the gluteus minimus (that's a favorite spot, actually), but the pain may run down the leg, mimicking sciatica. Or a trigger point in the gluteus medius may read as pain in the lower back. There are a lot of variations, but the patterns are well known and predictable, so professionals know where to look for the originating problem. Most of the time, anyway. Pretty soon, you will, too.

One thing that helps is that trigger point or muscle pain *in general* is recognizably different from nerve pain (again, this means pain in which an aggravated nerve is the source of the pain, not just the means of transmission to your brain) and other pain, so that you know what you are dealing with. Most of the time, nerve pain, for example, is "burning, sharp, electric," and you can pinpoint exactly where it is. Trigger point pain, on the other hand, is achy, diffuse, hard to localize, and dull. And it often arises far from the source, which is a trigger point in a muscle.

One reason it is called trigger point pain is that it is usually "triggered" by an actual event, just the way it feels. You rolled over funny in bed, you opened the Sub-Zero too vigorously, you picked up the box of books with your back, not your legs. Sometimes, those triggering events are one-off incidents, which is the way they feel. But more often, the trigger point (or vulnerability) has been building for a long time. Vulnerable muscles or muscle segments have been under repetitive pressure for a long time, and they are ready to "go" at the drop of a hat. You open the Sub-Zero funny and *pow*! A terrifying spasm. A latent trigger point like that can "go" without any trigger event at all or with a trifling one. Let us hope that yours is a "one-off," not one that has been building for years, because the one-off takes less time to heal. But never mind, the approach is just the same.

The most common trigger points are the ones that have been caused by muscular overload, and that have developed over time. Think of the familiar situation: You sit at your desk for months and years. It is an "unnatural" position, and it puts repetitive pressure on muscles that aren't built for it. Or it can be repetitively misplaced loads, caused by you doing some move the same wrong way, year after year, like a faulty golf swing. Say you sprain an ankle and you never quite rehab the ankle the way you should. Over the following weeks and months you walk slightly differently than you used to. This subtle change causes muscles in your legs and pelvis to bear loads in a different way. Some now bear more loads, some less. Over time, those muscles that are now bearing more loads get stressed and strained, and trigger points develop. The pain from these can come on gradually or suddenly. As we have said all along, most of the time, you have built your own back pain, over time, with the way you behave. That is true for most muscle pain, too.

## Finding Trigger Points

Okay, on to the details.

"For low back pain sufferers, the most important and common areas for trigger points to occur are in the lumbar paraspinals, quadratus lumborum, gluteus maximus, gluteus medius, gluteus minimus, and piriformis." Sorry, that's Jeremy; he just can't help himself. But you don't have to memorize the names; you just have to look at the pictures to get the general idea. And then feel around for the real source of the pain. When I say look at the pictures, I mean look and see if you can relate what you feel to the typical patterns the pictures show. The Xs represent the location of the *real* trigger point and the red shaded areas represent the area where you may *perceive* the pain. So think about where you *feel* the pain. Then look at the pictures. Then go

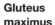

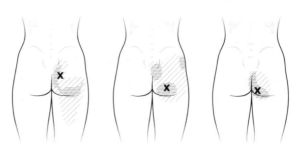

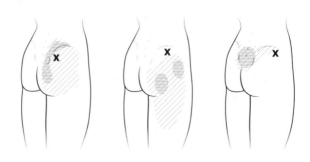

to work to find where the *X may* mark the spot. When you find it, it will hurt a lot more than the surrounding area. *Bingo!* Think of these pictures as "treasure maps" and the treasure is eventual release from pain.

This process is very much "hands on." It can be challenging to distinguish areas of perceived pain from actual trigger points until you get a feel for what you are looking for. If you try multiple times and fail, you may need the assistance of a good chiropractor, massage therapist, or physical therapist to get the

**Gluteus minimis**  **Piriformis**

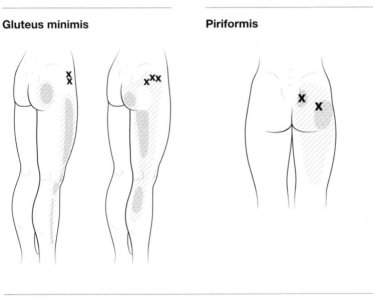

**Quadratus lumborum**

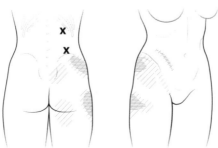

hang of this. To get started, grope around with your hands (using the pictures as a guide to the general area) until you have a fair idea of where the *real* trigger points are. You will know them because they hurt more. For once, the pain is the good news. It means that you're getting close. Or you're there.

By the way, the muscles where the trigger point lies can be deep. The gluteus minimus, for example, is buried beneath two other muscles and a layer of fat. Some of you are not going to have the strength or leverage to reach that trigger point with your hand alone. You may need to use a tennis ball or foam roller, which will be discussed in the following pages. But, to start, just use your hand until you get a general idea if there is something deep in those muscles that needs to be released. And don't forget: Use the pictures as your guide.

Once you have a general idea of where the trigger point is, mash away at it, if you like, with your bare hands, and see if that manual manipulation is enough to "release" the rascal. What you do is hold down hard on the place that hurts the most and—in ten to thirty seconds or so—you should feel an easing of the pain. That is the trigger point letting go. Nice work. If the pain does not ease up after thirty seconds or so, either you are not directly on the trigger point (move around very subtly and see if it's more intense just to the side of where you currently are) or this may not be a trigger point you are dealing with. If the pain gets worse as you stay on it and then continues to get worse when you let go, it could be a muscle tear, bursitis (the result of an inflamed sac, called a bursa), or worse. As we said, this challenge is tricky and if you struggle with it, get some help in the beginning. Often, however, you are going to need a gadget—not just your hands—to release the trigger point, once you find it.

# Finding and Releasing Gluteal Trigger Points with Assistant Device

Let's assume that you have traced your trigger point to somewhere in your glutes, which is a very common area to find it, but you have not had any luck releasing it with your bare hands. You need help. Look at the next set of pictures. These folks are using a simple tennis ball, which does remarkably well. You try it. Jeremy will walk you through.

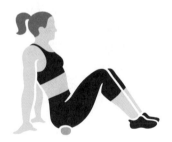 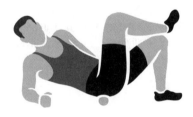

**Step 1:** Okay, sit on the floor, and grab a tennis ball.

**Step 2:** Place the tennis ball on the floor and slowly lower one side of your buttocks onto it, near where you think the trigger point lies. Try not to put your full weight onto it yet (it'll hurt too much).

**Step 3:** As always, brace your core.

**Step 4:** Gently roll back and forth until you feel a surprisingly tender spot. That, we hope, is a trigger point. It is not uncommon for these spots to refer pain down the leg or into the low back, but stick with the most tender spot.

**Step 5:** Once you find a sore spot, slowly lower your full body weight onto it if you can tolerate it. Breathe.

**Step 6:** As you exhale, try to relax the muscles in your buttocks. Your body is not going to want to let you do this;

your instinct is to tighten up because of the pain. Ignore your instincts, for once.

**Step 7:** If you are directly on a trigger point, the pain will be great. *But you will feel a slight lessening of the intensity of the pain in ten to thirty seconds.* Remember to breathe and relax each time you exhale. And congratulations. You've done it. Started to, anyway; it's going to take more than once, but you are there. When the pain eases, it is because you are literally releasing the spasm in the muscle. Nice.

**Step 8:** If you don't feel that lessening of pain, you might not be right on the trigger point. Roll around in very small circles (trigger points are *no bigger than a dime*) until you feel the most intense spot, and try again.

**Step 9:** Slowly move around again until you feel another trigger point. Repeat the steps.

**Step 10:** Some of you will notice that your chronic back pain is already noticeably diminished after doing this one time. That's a great sign! But you're not done. It does mean that your recovery is in sight. But you are going to have to do this more than once. And you're going to have to follow the rest of the instructions in this book about the long-term exercise regimen. The immediate relief can be so great that you are tempted to say, "I'm done." You are not done.

# Lower Back Trigger Points

Same story, but this time it's for folks whose trigger points seem to be in the lower back. Okay, here's Jeremy again.

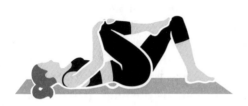 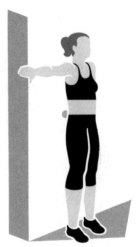

**Step 1:** You can do this lying on the floor or standing against a wall.

**Step 2:** Place a tennis ball under you on the muscles of your lower back on either side of the spine.

**Step 3:** Just as with the gluteal trigger points, gently roll around until you feel a very tender spot that may or may not radiate pain to another area.

**Step 4:** Whether lying down or standing, gently put more of your body weight into the trigger point.

**Step 5:** Use your breath to get this done. Try consciously to relax the muscle under the ball as you exhale. Doing this will allow you to get deeper into the muscle, targeting parts of the muscle you would not otherwise be able to reach.

**Step 6:** You should feel a noticeable lessening of the pain in ten to thirty seconds. If you don't, you may not be right on the trigger point. Roll around in very small circles (remember, trigger points are no bigger than a dime) until you feel the most intense spot, and try again.

## TROUBLESHOOTING FOR GLUTES AND LOWER BACK

See if any of the following complaints sound familiar.

- "I can't find any spots that hurt." If after multiple attempts at covering every square centimeter of the muscles in the glutes or low back you cannot find a spot that hurts intensely, congratulations! You don't have any trigger points. Move on to the next chapter.

- "The pain gets much worse, not better, as I hold pressure on it." If this occurs, one of two things is happening: You are on an area other than a trigger point or you aren't in the center of the trigger point. If the pain rapidly increases in intensity and lingers for a while after you release the pressure, you could be hitting a nerve or bursa. Avoid that area and move on. If the pain stays the same or increases just a little bit, you may not be directly on the center of the trigger point. Move around millimeter by millimeter and see if you can get a release.

- Again, some of you simply may not be able to do this. Go to a competent chiropractor or physical therapist and get a hand.

## CHAPTER FIFTEEN

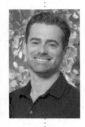

## RULE #6

# Crawl Before You Walk, Walk Before You Run

**From Jeremy**

A s you know by now, the essence of the protocol is life-long behavioral change. That means changing the way you carry yourself and move (the neutral spine and all that). But it also means adopting and staying with our carefully designed (and progressive) exercise regimen. It is designed for back pain and it is essential for a *permanent* cure. And you have to do it correctly. There is an awful lot of text and a bunch of pictures about exercise in this book. But it's not because you have to do so many exercises; there really aren't that many. It's because we want you to *do them right*. Remember, you are far more likely to do these exercises with the compensatory patterns you have been doing for years unless you read closely and concentrate on doing them the right way. Doing them the wrong way will just make you better at doing bad things.

One great key to doing them right is to go slow in the learning process. Whether you're the type or not, you have to take it step-by-step. This is a healing *process*, and you cannot rush a healing process; it has its own rhythm and you have to follow it. Roll out these exercises slowly over time, progressing from one level to the next only when you "get" the level you are on and are ready to move up.

Remember, it is these daily exercises that—more than anything else—are going to give most of you a significant *and permanent* reduction in pain and tightness. Other steps get you past the immediate pain. These steps make the change permanent.

## Be Still to Heal; Be Still to Stay Well

One of the main goals of changing your movement patterns is to make the "be still to heal" concept (Rule #2, in Chapter 7) part of your daily life. Once you have achieved an initial fix, you don't have to be *as still*. But it is a great idea to learn to move with relative stillness (without moving your lumbar spine too much) *all* the time.

This is a big change for most of you, and you have to take it in steps; as I say, you have to crawl before you walk. The first step in learning to keep your lumbar spine still *routinely* is simply to learn to march in place, with a neutral spine. (This is the "crawl" part of the process; it may seem too easy to bother with. It is not.) The goal is to learn to march in place with no lower spine movement. Then you can move on to other movements in this chapter.

*Key tip:* If any of these movements hurt, take a step back to the last thing you could do without pain (marching in place, for instance). Stay with that for a few more days and then try to progress again. In theory, if you can march in place without pain, you can walk without pain and move without pain. It's just a matter of building up your core, turning on the right muscles, and learning to use those muscles to move in the right way.

Whenever you have difficulty, go back to the previous step and start again.

Okay, you've done marching in place without moving your lower spine. Once that feels relatively simple, try doing this while walking. Things become a little murkier here because there are many factors at play. Because you are now weight-bearing, you need the support of important muscle groups like the glutes and latissimus dorsi (lats) to support your spine, in addition to the muscles we talked about in the core. If you can't do this at first without pain, follow the advice in the book for a while, and it will come once you have developed enough strength to support your spine while standing.

# Walking with Neutral Spine

Learning to walk with a neutral spine means applying the same mechanics of your Slow March with Neutral Spine exercise (page 94) to an upright, weight-bearing position. Almost everyone can improve their ability to walk without pain if they can do the slow march exercise on the ground. The distance you can walk without pain, or without significant increases in pain, will increase as you build core and gluteal strength and endurance by doing the exercises in this book. To get started on increasing your ability to walk with decreased pain, follow these directions:

**Step 1:** Stand with good posture. Stand tall, shoulders back, head over your shoulders. Think of sticking your chest out and pulling your shoulder blades down and back. Make sure you aren't leaning forward. Tilt your pelvis back and forth (just like you did on the floor earlier), and stop where your lower back feels the most comfortable.

**Step 2:** Use your core to lock your neutral spine in place.

**Step 3:** Now try to walk while maintaining the position of your lower back and with the good posture you just set. It can help to put one hand on your stomach and one on your low back to feel for movement. Once you feel like you've mastered maintaining neutral spine while walking, start to swing your arms from the shoulders, arm to opposite leg. This means if your right leg is swinging forward, your left arm should be as well. Make sure to always swing your arms from the shoulders as you walk; this helps dissipate force away from the spine. This movement takes time to master so don't get frustrated. Keep practicing. It gets easier after you have built endurance and strength in the muscles that support the spine.

**Step 4:** If you sense your back is about to hurt, stop and have a seat for a few minutes and give your back a break. Then try walking a little longer. Over time, the period between these sitting breaks should increase, allowing you to walk farther without pain.

Now let's move on to more complex movements. To make it easier (and to improve your chances of success) we are going to break those more complex movements down into pieces and then put them all together at the end. We will start with *movement from the hips*, a very basic move in all our lives all the time. Let's start with hip-hinging. Hip-hinging is a way to bend forward without stressing (i.e., bending) the spine. Done right, the axis of movement is in the hips, not the low back. Your low back should be in a protected neutral position with the core engaged. As you bend forward, your low back doesn't round or move. Let's look at a picture of hip-hinging and a picture of lumbar flexion (low back bending); one is good, the other is bad. This is simple stuff, but it is very hard to get over your ancient, bad habits. Hard but essential.

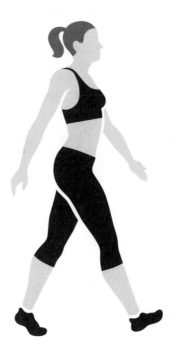

# Hip-Hinge with Neutral Spine

Here are a couple of pictures showing you the right way to hinge (on the left) and the wrong way (on the right). Notice the very slightly curved lower back in the hip-hinge picture on the left: *no movement.* Excellent! The pic on the right has quite a lot of spine movement; don't do that. When you first try this movement, it may feel awkward, and you may assume that you cannot reach as far forward with good posture. Not so. You'll soon realize that you can move just as far forward, using only your hips, as you did before, using your back. You don't lose anything and you avoid a ton of pain. Over time you will gain mobility. The reason is that moving with your lower back eventually causes pain and stiffness in your back. But moving from your hips will not have that result. Let's practice doing it right.

RIGHT     WRONG

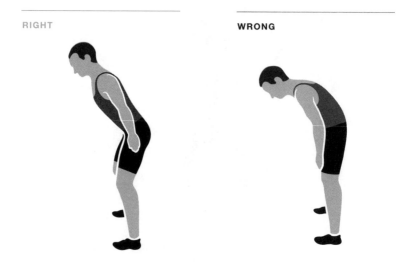

**Step 1:** Stand with feet shoulder-width apart.

**Step 2:** Set your posture: Find neutral spine, brace the core, shoulders back, stand as tall as you can without pain and without breaking neutral spine.

**Step 3:** Bend your knees slightly.

**Step 4:** Feel the two bones sticking out of the sides of your hips. These are called your greater trochanters. Picture a pole going through these two points, passing right through your pelvis. This is your imaginary axis of movement.

**Step 5:** Now place one hand on your stomach and the other on your back. On your back, put your fingers on those little bones sticking out (spinous processes). You are putting your hands here to feel for any unwanted movement when you hip-hinge.

**Step 6:** Without moving anything in the core (you shouldn't feel those little bones in your back moving), slowly bend forward on that imaginary axis of movement through the hip bones while sticking your buttocks out behind you a little bit. If you feel your stomach or back move, stop, reset, and try again.

**Step 7:** Go only as far forward as you can without moving your back. For many of you, your hamstrings (back of legs) are going to be a limiting

factor in your range of motion in the beginning. Don't worry if you can't go too far. Your hamstrings will loosen up in time if you follow all of the advice in this book.

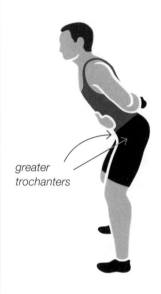

*greater trochanters*

**Step 8:** Slowly return to the starting position without moving your back or stomach.

**Step 9:** This should not hurt your low back. If it does, reset your stance, find neutral spine, brace your core. Not hurting? Now try it again with a very small range of motion. Stay within the range of motion that doesn't hurt. Slowly increase your range of motion over time—it will come.

## Adding Rotation

Now let's get a little more complex. Let's add rotation to the bend. Hip-hinging correctly allows you to move forward and backward without pain. Now let's learn to move side to side. We are talking rotation. Again, think about moving from the hips. It's easiest to visualize proper rotation if you think about your waist. We don't want any movement at the waist. Try to picture your rib cage being locked on to your pelvis. That's what you want. Pretend that there are no joints between your ribs and pelvis, for this one.

# Full-Body Rotation

The chest, navel, and hips all move together. This means there is no (or very little) movement in the spine. The body rotates by moving the hips, knees, and pelvis. If the hips and pelvis stay facing forward while the rib cage moves, the movement comes from the waist, and therefore the lumbar spine. This type of movement can wear down the discs and joints in the spine over time, especially when additional load is applied (like unloading the dishwasher for instance). Just like hip-hinging, rotation done properly doesn't cause you to lose mobility and will improve athletic performance. Let's give it a try. Once again, the new movement is not that hard. But you are trying to unlearn a life-time of moving with your spine. That *is* hard.

**Step 1:** Stand with your feet shoulder-width apart.

**Step 2:** Set your posture: Find neutral spine, brace the core, shoulders back, stand as tall as you can without pain and without breaking neutral spine.

**Step 3:** Bend your knees slightly.

**Step 4:** Place your hands on the top of your pelvis with your fingers pointed forward. This hand position is to help you visualize movement of the pelvis as you get used to this movement.

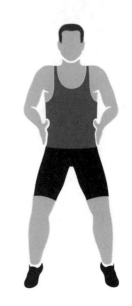

**Step 5:** Keep the knees bent and loose but the core engaged, and try to turn a little to the right by shifting the knees and hips. Your fingers, navel, hip bones, chest bone, and face should all point the same direction. It's okay if you pivot the feet a little bit.

**Step 6:** Now try to the left.

**Step 7:** Slowly increase your range of motion by bending more at the knees.

**Step 8:** Then increase your range of motion even more by pivoting your feet.

**Step 9:** At all times and especially at the end of the movement, your chest bone, head, navel, and hips should be in alignment.

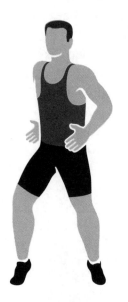 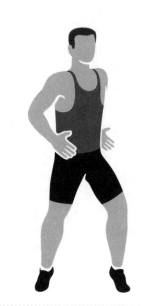

## TROUBLESHOOTING

Knee pain: Stay lighter on your feet and pivot the ball of the inside foot (the side you are moving away from) as you rotate.

# Torso Rotation with Hip-Hinge and Squat

Now let's try to put those two movements—the hip-hinge and the rotation—together with a squat for a realistic, three-dimensional movement that allows you to accomplish everyday tasks (think unloading the dishwasher, putting up groceries) without stressing your back. You are going to rotate and bend down (hip-hinge), then come back up to the other side and extend.

Notice that within that entire chain of movement, the person in the drawing does not really move his spine (look at the waist if you're having trouble visualizing that). The rib cage remains locked onto the pelvis the entire time. These pictures show you that you can go almost 180 degrees from side to side, stooping as low as you can and then extending as high as your hands can go, without compromising your back. Let's try it.

**Step 1:** Stand with your feet shoulder-width apart.

**Step 2:** Find neutral spine and engage your core to lock it in.

**Step 3:** Stand with good posture.

**Step 4:** Rotate torso to the right without twisting the waist as before.

**Step 5:** Pivot the inside foot (left foot, in this case) as you turn.

**Step 6:** After initiating the rotation, start to hinge at the hips, bending forward. Remember not to round your back.

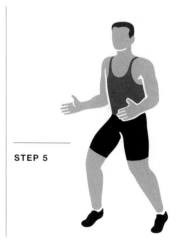

STEP 5

**Step 7:** Go only as low and as far to the right as you can without twisting at the waist or rounding your low back. You will now be in a squat/split squat position.

**Step 8:** Reach out with your arms as if you were picking something up off of the floor.

**Step 9:** Bring the arms back in and re-center your weight over your buttocks and feet.

**Step 10:** Using your glutes, lift yourself out of the lowered position, pushing with your right glutes as you rotate back to midline while hinging back up through the hips.

**Step 11:** As you swing past midline (without twisting at the waist!), pivot your right foot, continuing to use the right glutes, and extend your arms up toward the ceiling as if you were putting something on a shelf.

**Step 12:** Return to the starting position without twisting at the waist. Try this in front of a mirror several times.

**Step 13:** Then try this movement on the opposite side of your body.

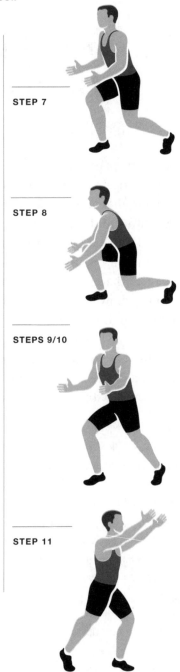

STEP 7

STEP 8

STEPS 9/10

STEP 11

## TROUBLESHOOTING

- Knee pain: If your knees hurt as you start to rotate the torso, be lighter on your feet. Allow the feet to pivot a little bit. If the knees hurt when you are hinged forward at the bottom of the movement, drop your buttocks back more so that you are in a squat position (think of a baseball catcher) and lessen your range of motion. Try doing small movements and increase your range of motion gradually.

- Back pain: If your back hurts with this one, it is likely you are twisting at the waist, rounding the back, or don't have the gluteal strength yet to perform this movement to its full range of motion. Do a little investigating: Can you hip-hinge without pain? If so, that's not the issue. Can you do the torso rotation without pain? Can you squat without pain? If you can do all three without pain then it is likely you are having difficulty putting all of these moves together without sacrificing form on one of them. Try doing this movement in very small pieces in front of a mirror or loved one, and gradually increase your range of motion over time. If any one piece causes pain, work on that one until you can do it pain-free, and then come back and try this movement again.

Remember, these movements must become habits. That sounds daunting but it really isn't that hard. Once your back starts to feel better, it will let you know when you move the wrong way and you'll avoid that at all costs.

## CHAPTER SIXTEEN

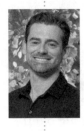

## RULE #7

# Stand Tall for the Long Haul

**From Jeremy**

ealing your back is a lifelong commitment, and it isn't easy. But it's a lot easier than living with back pain.

We've been through most of it, now. You've learned to keep your spine stable. You've learned how to build up your core so it has the strength to hold a neutral spine as a default position throughout the day. And you've learned to work on your strength generally. Excellent. But there's this one last step: integrating what you've learned into your daily life. Do not be impatient with this part; true behavioral change takes time and repetition. It may take months—and reading this book more than once—before sound posture and movements become second nature. I just want to show you some practical applications of everything you've learned so far.

At the end of this chapter, I will talk about how to find a good physical therapist or chiropractor if you need one from time to time. We are most assuredly not giving up on you. It's just that we know there are a couple of steps in this chapter that some of you will find challenging, and getting a little help is not cheating.

## Sitting

You spend a lot of time sitting, so you will want to *do it right!* Let it be part of the healing process, not part of the problem. Ideal sitting posture looks like the person's on the right. Bad posture looks like the person's on the left.

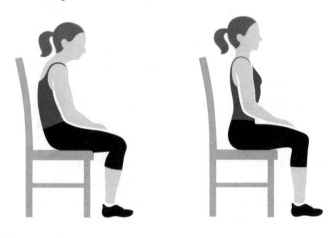

Your "sits" bones (actually called ischial tuberosities, those pointy bones you can feel under your buttocks when you sit) should be under your shoulders with a slight curve in the low back (or whatever your neutral spine may be). The knees should be at a 70-degree angle, with your feet on the floor under you or slightly in front of you. Your head should be over your shoulders (not forward) with your shoulders back and down. This is the ideal position for short bouts of sitting. Why just short bouts? Because short bouts is all the sitting you should do. The *great secret of sitting is this: Don't do too much of it! You should not sit still for more than twenty to thirty minutes at a stretch.* Then get up and do something, if only for *thirty* seconds, to stop the *creep. Move!*

## AT THE OFFICE

For those of you who work at a desk with a computer, the posture on the right is the ideal posture, for short bouts of time.

You want your elbows to be close to a 90-degree angle and the screen positioned so that your head looks naturally forward while sitting squarely on your shoulders. If you work on a laptop or tablet, I strongly suggest you use it on a desk instead of your lap. If you work exclusively on a tablet, get a keyboard for it and put the tablet on a stand when you plan to work on it for a while. (Though if you have neck or back issues, a desktop computer is a better choice than a tablet or laptop.) Another strong recommendation is to alternate between sitting and standing, with an adjustable standing desk if possible. This position shifts the potentially harmful loads that can accumulate throughout the day to different parts of your body, and prevents overload in one particular area. I don't recommend going from eight hours per day of sitting to eight hours per day of standing, because this can cause a host of other problems that are not just related to your back. Go back and forth throughout the day.

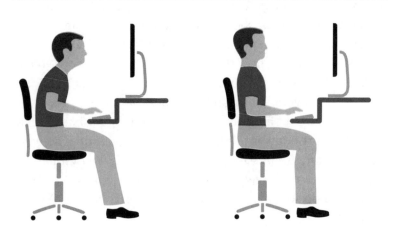

## SMARTPHONES

There are a few great terms coined by others to describe a recent phenomenon in spine care. "Text neck" and "iHunch" are a few favorites. We are now literally seeing X-rays taken of kids age twelve to fifteen that show as much spinal degeneration as the X-rays of a sixty year-old! This is because of the all-too-common sight in the picture below: a kid curled attentively around his iPhone. Or a grown-up, come to think of it.

Smartphones are a catastrophe for our necks and backs. Why? Remember *creep*? Keeping your neck and back bent in the same position for an extended time strains the muscles and ligaments and eventually causes joint degeneration. Other than drastically cutting back on your phone or tablet usage, there is no easy solution. But here are a few suggestions.

First, of course, just try to limit the amount of time you spend emailing and web surfing on your smartphone. Do your best to save these activities for your computer, where it is easier to maintain good posture. Or use your smartphone when you are sitting in a better position. This is tricky because it is automatic

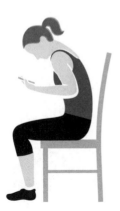 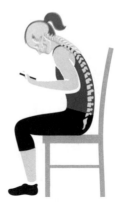

to hold it out in front of you (like the person in the picture), look down, and raise hell with your neck and back. But you can try. Try lying on a couch, for example, with the phone over your head. Dunno if you can do that all day long but it sure is better for your back. Or lie on your side with the phone in front of you. Or change the position of your phone or tablet every few minutes. Hold it up in front of your face, move it to the side, stop for a minute and look around, etc. You're smart or you wouldn't be reading our book: Just think of something. We realize you're not going to give up your smartphone, but you're not going to change nature, either. So, when you use your smartphone, figure out a way to do it with a neutral spine! Be a model to your kids. And save your own back!

# Getting Out of a Chair

Getting out of a chair is just doing the second part of a squat—the rising part. This also applies to getting off of the toilet and any other related movements. Have a seat in a chair in which your feet are near the ground or on the ground when you are seated. Follow these steps to perform a squat out of the chair. Make this a habit and do it every time you get up.

**Step 1:** Slide forward so that your sits bones (the bones you can feel in your buttocks when you sit) are at the edge of the chair.

**Step 2:** Find neutral spine and brace your core to lock it in place.

**Step 3:** Hinge forward at the hips so that your low back doesn't move,

and put your feet on the floor. See (in the picture) how this is the same as the first part of the squat when you hip-hinged to stick your buttocks out behind you? As you start to shift your weight from the chair onto your feet, start to "spread the floor"/ "tear the piece of paper" (pages 160–161) to engage the glutes as you rise.

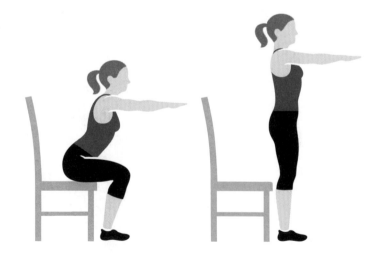

**Step 4:** Bring the hips up and forward as you squeeze the glutes to come into a standing position, all while maintaining neutral spine and abdominal brace.

**Step 5:** Try this several times until you feel the glutes doing most of the work.

**Step 6:** Can you picture how this translates to getting out of the car, off the toilet, etc.? We hope so.

# Getting Up off the Floor

The split squat, once you master it, can be a great way to get up off the floor without aggravating your back. Here's how.

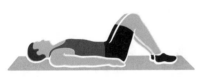

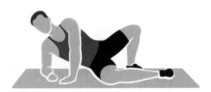

**Step 1:** Start in any position on the floor.

**Step 2:** Turn over to your hands and knees.

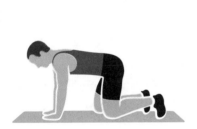

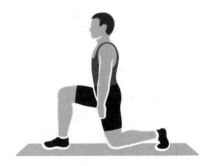

**Step 3:** Find your neutral spine and engage your core to lock it in.

**Step 4:** Come into a half-kneeling position, with one leg forward and bent at a 90-degree angle while you kneel on the back leg.

**Step 5:** Come up onto the ball of your back foot.

**Step 6:** You are now at the bottom of the split squat position (page 163). Rise up from this position using the glutes of the rear leg just as you did in the split squat.

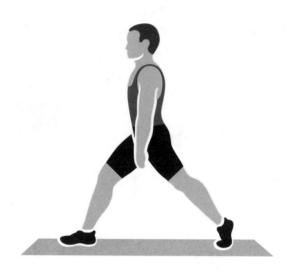

This can be difficult at first. Practice the split squat and get good at it before you attempt this. With time, this movement becomes a great way to get off the floor without hurting your back or knees.

# Lifting

As most of you know by now, picking up heavy objects (and not so heavy objects) can be risky if you have back problems. Depending on your personal condition, you may not be able to get back to picking up heavy objects for a while. Or ever. But most of you will get back to it in time (up to fifty pounds or so, depending). When you do pick things up, of whatever weight, there are some things you can do to reduce the risk.

**Step 1:** *Shorten the lever arm between you and the object.* By lever arm, I mean the distance between you and the object at the time that you start to lift it off of the ground. Whenever possible, pull the object in close to the body before you start to lift it upward.

**Step 2:** *Use your glutes as much as possible.* Remember, these big strong muscles are designed to help you lift things. If you aren't using the glutes, you are compensating with much smaller, weaker muscles that are more likely to become overwhelmed.

Follow the squat directions when lifting.

**Step 3:** *If you have to rotate, move your feet instead of twisting your torso.* If you can't move your feet, practice the good rotational patterns taught in Chapter 15.

**Step 4:** *Always keep your neutral spine and a strong core brace.* When lifting a heavy object you may need a bit more of a core contracting than normal. But make sure not to confuse this with "sucking in" or "bearing down," since that will increase abdominal pressure and can put more stress on the discs.

Also, you can refer back to the Torso Rotation with Hip-Hinge and Squat (page 187).

## Household Activities

These are the sneaky little day-to-day activities that can really cause big problems, in my experience. Most people think that if something isn't heavy they don't have to move or lift in a spine-healthy manner. This is anything but true. Remember geologic time? Doing these simple, seemingly harmless activities day in and day out are like the wind against a solid rock. Do them often enough and, over time, they will cause real damage. Common activities in this category include vacuuming, unloading the dishwasher, putting away groceries, mowing the lawn, picking up your kids, shoveling snow, pulling weeds, and sitting on the couch. Do those things correctly: Think about all the lessons in the book, every time you reach down to pick something up.

## Driving

The same rules apply to driving as sitting, with one exception: People tend to lean with their right foot forward when they drive in order to use the pedals. If you do a lot of driving, this can eventually cause a subtle shift in the pelvis. An unbalanced pelvis can lead to back pain. Do your best to sit symmetrically when driving, but remember, if you are sitting for more than twenty or thirty minutes it's best to move around and change positions so you aren't putting too much load on one small area in your back. If you are on a long drive, stop and get out of the car at least every hour to minimize the effects of creep. And a lumbar support pillow can be a lifesaver if driving bothers your back.

## Sleeping

Sleeping can be a huge challenge. Let's start with mattress selection. If you have back pain as soon as you get up in the morning, chances are your mattress is playing a role. Try experimenting with different mattresses to see if the pattern changes. (I know this isn't easy, but it is worth the time and effort. For some people, a change in mattress can be the biggest factor in permanent back pain relief.) Go sleep in a hotel or a guest bedroom or a child's bedroom. Is your back pain any different when you wake up? Better? Worse? If it is in any way different, then it is very likely that your mattress is playing some role in your back pain. There is no rigid rule to follow, but the following is usually true: Those who are skinny tend to do best on firm mattresses while those who are less so tend to do better on a softer mattress. This is because those body type/firmness combos allow the spine to stay relatively neutral. Again, this won't apply to everyone but it can give you some guidance. There are now companies out there that are making mattresses specifically for back pain. Some of them are quite good.

Regarding sleeping position, the best for most people is on your back. Unfortunately most people can't sleep like this. In my experience most of the other positions have their benefits and negatives based on each individual person. Try to find what works best for you with one exception: If you find that you are stiff in the low back in the morning and you feel bent forward, it is likely that you have tight psoas muscles. These are the big hip flexors that connect from the front of your spine to your thighs. If this is the case, you want to *avoid sleeping in the fetal position* with your knees bent. This shortens the psoas throughout the night, making them tighter. So stretch out.

## Sex

This subject is a delicate one, but we want to cover it because it's very important for happiness and well-being and because there are real techniques that can help you have an active sex life without hurting your back. If you've been following this book closely you can probably figure it out yourself. Can you guess? You have to keep a neutral spine and practice hip-hinging. This can be challenging with the movements involved in sexual intercourse. Feedback from my patients and my knowledge of biomechanics tell me that the easiest position in which to accomplish this, for both partners is "doggie style," with the partner on all fours maintaining neutral spine and core brace and the kneeling partner with neutral spine, hinging at the hips. Awfully sorry to intrude on your private life like this (I'm embarrassed, too), but—if you can bear this position—it is much easier to hip-hinge while kneeling than while lying down. Just like all other activities, sex will become easier once your back pain has calmed down from practicing the strategies we have given you in this book. (Then, as Chris said, reading this chapter, "You can get back to your good old animal self.")

## Finding a Good Physical Therapist or Chiropractor

As I mentioned in Chapter 14 when talking about trigger points, it may be necessary in the short term to find a good physical therapist to help you with some of this. Also, for a small number of the most difficult cases, you may need long-term care from a skilled clinician. If you can't make it out to Aspen, I hope this can help you find someone nearby. Like finding a good mattress, there is no easy rule to follow, but I've developed some tips that should be helpful. In addition, we hope to implement a test that therapists must pass if they want to advertise on our website. So those who advertise with us will have gone through at least a rough screen of competence. Otherwise, try these "rules" for finding a physical therapist.

1. Referrals from someone you trust are best.

2. Be wary of chiropractors who try to lock you in to multiple (ten or more) visits at once, especially if they don't mention exercise or behavior modification early in your treatment program.

3. Be wary of chiropractors and physical therapists who only do manual therapy with no mention of habits, posture, movement, and so on, after a few sessions. It may be necessary for them to perform manual therapy only the first few times, but a discussion on behavior and exercise should happen at least in the first week or two.

4. A good physical therapist or chiropractor will likely ask you about your habits and activities of daily life and suggest that you alter or limit some of them in the short term until the pain gets better.

5. A good therapist (chiropractor or physical therapist) will always take a good, detailed history and ask you probing questions to assess your condition. In addition, the therapist should almost always perform some tests to pinpoint the pain-generating tissue.

6. If you have pain in the buttock or leg, a good therapist will ask questions about that and will determine whether this is

a nerve problem. These questions should include whether or not you have experienced numbness, tingling, or strength loss. If the answer to any of those questions is yes, the therapist should either perform a neurological exam or ask whether you have had one recently.

7. A good therapist will spend more than five to ten minutes with you if they are trying to eradicate chronic back pain. It just cannot be done in that amount of time. There are some cases where acute back pain can be treated with a quick adjustment, but not *chronic* pain.

## CHAPTER SEVENTEEN

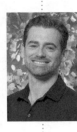

# Mobility Where It Matters

**From Jeremy**

We have talked an awful lot about being "still" and maintaining stability. What about mobility, which is more or less the opposite of stillness? I get asked this a lot. For low back pain sufferers, the place in which you want to promote flexibility and mobility is in the hips and lower extremities. This short chapter teaches you how to increase and maintain flexibility in the muscles and mobility in the joints in the hips and lower extremities. These few exercises should be done every day. They will add only a minute or two to your workout time.

A lack of flexibility in the big muscles of the lower extremities and lack of mobility in the hip joints will cause increased pressure and load on the lumbar spine while limiting blood flow to important areas. Maintaining flexibility and mobility requires a combination of dynamic mobilization exercises and static stretching.

## Mobilizations

When we refer to maintaining range of motion in a joint, we use the term "mobility." This is not a stretch but rather a movement where the goal is to move the joint through its maximum range of motion without compromising the low back. For our purposes, hip mobility is the most important. As we have said throughout the book, we want to maximize movement in the hips while minimizing movement in the lumbar spine.

Aside from the effects of limited hip mobility on the low back, it is also important to maintain hip mobility for the health of the hip itself. The hip joint has no direct blood supply and therefore relies on the pressure generated by movement in the joint to "squeeze" nutrients (synovial fluid) into the joint space. The more limited your range of motion in the hip, the less synovial fluid is "squeezed" in and the hip will eventually suffer and degenerate. This can ultimately lead to a hip replacement and other operations. We promote maximum hip mobility by lengthening the muscles around the hip through stretching and by performing mobilization exercises to "oil" the hip joint.

# Hip Circles

This movement is an important mobilization. Do this one before you exercise.

**Step 1:** Get on your hands and knees.

**Step 2:** Find neutral spine and brace your core.

**Step 3:** Lift one knee slightly and pretend to "draw" circles on the floor with your kneecap, getting maximum range of motion out of the hip joint without moving your low back. In other words, your hip joint should be performing all of the movement. Your back should not move at all. Done properly, you should feel your abdominal muscles working pretty hard to keep your back still while you do this movement.

**Step 4:** Do ten circles clockwise, ten counterclockwise, and then switch sides.

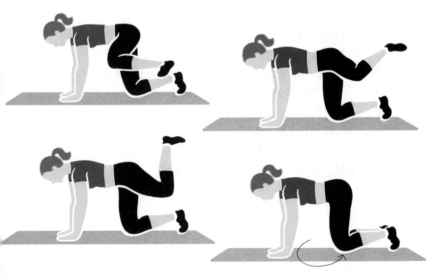

Don't arch the low back or hike your hip. Keep the low back still and in place.

## Stretches

In my experience, people tend to rely far too much on stretching when trying to heal their backs. Stretching has its place but must be done in combination with all of the other strategies (changing habits, spinal stabilization, strengthening the core) in this book. The more balanced and stable your spine and its related muscles become, the less you should need to stretch over time.

To increase flexibility in muscles, stretches need to be held for a good while, between forty-five and sixty seconds according to some research. The stretch also needs to be fairly intense to facilitate muscle lengthening. The stretches in this chapter are "static" stretches. Static stretches are held in place for long periods of time. These are done to promote muscle lengthening. These are not to be confused with "dynamic" stretches. Dynamic stretches are stretches that are performed with movement and are best done prior to exercises. The dynamic hamstring stretch in your daily routine is one example.

The key muscles to maintain flexibility are the hamstrings, glutes, piriformis, and psoas. For each of the following four stretches, try to hold for forty-five to sixty seconds with an intensity of about a 6/10. When performing the stretch, make sure that everything is relaxed except your arms, which are doing the work. Also maintain a light core brace to protect your back. Perform these stretches after exercise.

# Hamstring Stretch

**Step 1:** Get a belt, towel, or strap. It should about twice the length of your leg.

**Step 2:** Lie on your back. Place the strap around your foot.

**Step 3:** Find neutral spine and brace your core.

**Step 4:** Slowly pull one leg up until you feel a moderate stretch (about a 6/10 in intensity).

**Step 5:** Hold for forty-five to sixty seconds. Make sure your arms and core are the only parts of your body working. Everything else should be relaxed.

**Step 6:** Repeat on the other side.

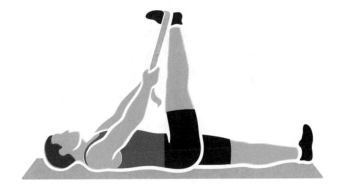

# Glute Stretch

**Step 1:** Lie on your back. Find neutral spine. Brace core lightly.

**Step 2:** Cross one leg over the other.

**Step 3:** Put your hands around the thigh of the uncrossed leg and use it as a lever to pull back the crossed leg, stretching the buttock.

**Step 4:** Hold for forty-five to sixty seconds. Make sure that your arms and core are the only areas working. Everything else should be relaxed.

**Step 5:** Repeat on other side.

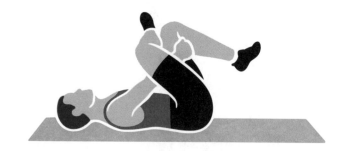

# Piriformis Stretch

**Step 1:** Lie on your back.

**Step 2:** Find neutral spine and brace your core. Bend one knee and bring it toward your chest.

**Step 3:** Grab the top/outside of the foot of the bent leg with the opposite hand as shown.

**Step 4:** With the other hand, grab the knee.

**Step 5:** Pull the knee to the opposite shoulder, creating a stretch in the buttock area.

**Step 6:** Hold for forty-five to sixty seconds. Make sure that your arms and core are the only areas working. Everything else should be relaxed.

**Step 7:** Repeat on other side.

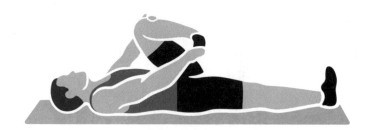

# Psoas Stretch

This stretch is slightly more difficult than the others. The goal is to feel a stretch in the top of the thigh, groin, and inside the abdominal wall.

**Step 1:** Get in a half-kneeling position: One leg will be in front of you, knee bent, and foot on the floor. The other leg will be below you, knee bent, with lower leg and knee resting on the floor.

**Step 2:** Find neutral spine and brace your core.

**Step 3:** Shift your body forward by "pointing" your hip bone straight out in front of you while simultaneously squeezing the glutes on that side. You should maintain neutral spine, not round your back or hinge forward at the hips.

**Step 4:** Bring your arms up over your head. You should feel the stretch in the thigh, groin, and/or inner abdomen. Hold for forty-five to sixty seconds. Then switch sides.

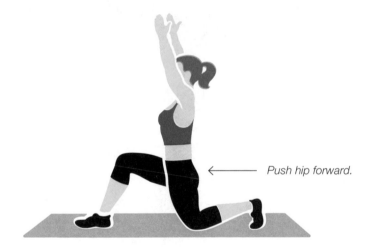

*Push hip forward.*

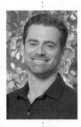

CHAPTER EIGHTEEN

# Special Conditions

.................................................................

**From Jeremy**

find this material fascinating but *you don't have to read it unless you have one of the headlined conditions*. This is an effort to give *some help* to people with serious conditions who are likely to need medical help, or at least some level of medical supervision as well as "book help."

There are some more extreme or special conditions causing back pain for which you are going to want to receive individual guidance from a physician but for which you may also get substantial help from the book. Here and elsewhere, you may ask: If I have to go to a therapist for this anyway, why not leave it all to him or her? The answer is twofold. First, the concepts and exercises in the book will give you a great foundation on which to build the more specific treatments suggested by your caregiver. But, second, in my experience, too many therapists treating these conditions jump right into the specific exercises and stretches for these conditions without building an adequate foundation of spine health and strength. That's what this book does.

So . . . get started with this book and then seek out specific treatment. But be alert: Some of these exercises can exacerbate pain for some sufferers. If that happens to you, stop. Sorry that this is so complicated. You are almost always going to get substantial help from the *general advice* you have already read but—for these special conditions—you will also benefit from the *specific advice* in this chapter. See your doctor and strike your own balance between medical help and the advice we offer here. It is a two-sided approach and—often with these special conditions—both can help. Typically, the medical help alone—great relief though it may be—is not going to provide a complete, permanent solution.

## Disc Herniations

This means a burst disc and it is very serious business, as you already know. You should start by seeing a medical doctor. If a doctor has told you that you should try conservative (that is, nonintrusive) care for a herniated disc but you are in too much pain to start this book, you may benefit from a steroid injection to calm the pain down. I am slow to recommend that step, but this may be one of the situations where it makes sense. Sometimes an injection can bring the pain and inflammation down to a tolerable level so that rehab exercises can be undertaken. You should be warned that steroid injections can slow the healing process of a herniated disc. Talk with your doctor about the risks and benefits of a steroid injection.

If you are having pain down your leg from a herniated disc, something called nerve *flossing* can sometimes help. It may sound like a joke, but it is not. Nerve flossing is a technique that attempts to traction or "scrub" the nerve roots as they exit the spinal cord near the herniated disc to remove material that sometimes builds up on them. If there is "stuff" stuck to the nerve roots or nerves (it is likely to be either pieces of disc material or scar tissue), that "stuff" can cause or exacerbate pain, and removing it can help a lot. Nerve flossing can sometimes do precisely that and provide significant relief. Caution: This technique can sometimes cause an increase in pain initially, before it reduces it. Sometimes it doesn't work. But it works enough to be worth the shot. There are countless YouTube videos out there on this subject. My favorite approach is Dr. Stuart McGill's. He has various videos and describes his approach in detail in his books.

## Hypermobile Sacroiliac (SI) Joint Pain

This pain can be one of the most difficult and stubborn conditions to treat, in my experience. The sacroiliac, or "SI," joint is the joint in your pelvis where the sides of your pelvis connect with your sacrum.

The SI joint is not supposed to move very much in a healthy individual. It is crossed by large ligaments and muscles that keep it taut. SI joints that move too much can cause recurring episodes of severe pain. This commonly starts with a sprain of these ligaments from a hard fall to the buttocks or from giving birth. Once the ligaments are deformed, the SI joint can become unstable. Learning to engage the core and gluteal muscles at the appropriate times can help people with chronic SI pain.

A medical intervention is sometimes needed. One approach is prolotherapy, an injection therapy whose goal is to tighten up loose ligaments and stabilize joints. An irritant is injected around the SI joint to cause scarring and stiffening of the ligaments that cross the joint, resulting in a more stable joint. In my experience, this works slightly more than 50 percent of the time.

Try this book first and see how much relief you get. You will likely get significant relief. If not, consult several prolotherapy practitioners before deciding to try it.

Before considering prolotherapy, try these exercises in addition to the ones you've already learned.

# Isometric Adduction

The goal here is to strengthen the muscles on the insides of your legs without moving the unstable SI joint. You will need a medicine ball, thick pillow, or something similar for this exercise.

**Step 1:** Lie on your back with your knees bent. Put the medicine ball between your knees.

**Step 2:** Find your neutral spine and brace your core.

**Step 3:** Squeeze the ball between the knees with 50 percent strength, being careful not to lose your core brace. Hold for ten seconds.

**Step 4:** Repeat ten reps. Do two to three sets.

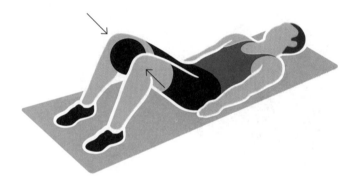

# Isometric Abduction

As with the previous exercise, the goal is to avoid moving the unstable SI joint. The difference here is that you are working on the muscles on the outside of your hips. You will need tubing or an elastic band for this exercise.

**Step 1:** Lie on your back with your knees bent.

**Step 2:** Find neutral spine and brace your core.

**Step 3:** Wrap the band or tube around your thighs and below the knees.

**Step 4:** Engage your glutes and move your knees outward about 45 degrees.

**Step 5:** Hold ten seconds.

**Step 6:** Do ten reps, two to three sets.

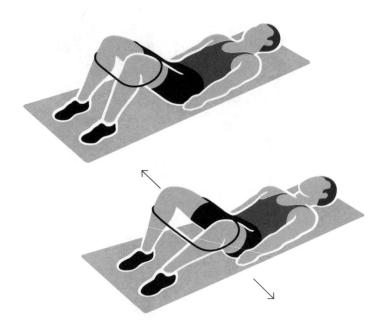

# "Bicycles" on Your Side

This exercise is very challenging to do properly. One of the goals is to keep your leg in the same "horizontal plane" throughout. By this I mean not to let your leg wander up or down if you were viewing it from the side. Rather, keep it steady with the knee and foot in the same position relative to each other throughout the movement.

**Step 1:** Lie on your side with your top arm on the floor in front of you for support.

**Step 2:** Brace your core.

**Step 3:** With the movement of bicycle pedaling in mind, raise your top knee up toward your torso and then push the foot out in front of you. Then bring it back behind you to make a big circle at the hip, as if you were pedaling a bicycle on your side. As you bring the leg behind you, focus on engaging the glutes and opening up the front of the hip.

**Step 4:** Go only as far as you can without moving your back.

**Step 5:** Do ten reps.

**Step 6:** Then, go the opposite direction.

**Step 7:** Push your heel back behind you, engaging the glutes and stretching out your hip flexors as your foot goes behind you.

**Step 8:** While moving the leg, do not let it wander up or down. In other words, stay in the same horizontal plane the entire time.

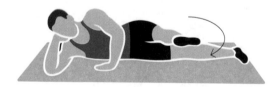

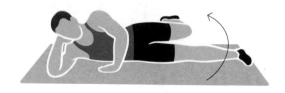

## Bulging Disc

Most bulging discs will heal on their own if pressures are taken off and the bulging disc is given the chance to recover. The most important thing with a bulging disc is to stop irritating it. You will need to limit activities that put the most pressure on the disc. This means doing much less of any activity that involves a seated position (driving, flying, etc.) as well as picking things up with a rounded back and twisting with the low back (golf, tennis, etc.). There are ways to continue to play these sports without twisting or bending the low back. Remember the concept of *creep* when you are required to sit. Break it up into twenty- to thirty-minute increments if you are required to sit all day. Avoiding *creep* is even more urgent when you have a bulging disc.

For some people, "press-ups" can help with bulging disc pain. These were initially recommended by Dr. Joseph McKenzie in his McKenzie protocol. His idea was that this exercise helps to shift the disc back into its natural position.

# Press-Ups

I have seen some people, but certainly not all people, benefit from this. But it is worth a try.

**Step 1:** Lie facedown on the floor with your elbows bent and your arms flat on the floor on either side of you, palms down.

**Step 2:** Lightly brace your core.

**Step 3:** Here's the hard part: You are going to attempt to press your upper body up off the floor *without* using the muscles in your low back. Your arms should be doing all of the work and your low back should be relaxed. If you have a bulging disc and you start to lift your torso up with your back muscles, there's a good chance they will go into spasm and make things quite a bit worse.

**Step 4:** Very slowly and very carefully, start to push your upper body up off the floor. If your low back muscles kick in, stop and slowly lower yourself back to the floor to start again.

**Step 5:** Continue up slowly. Go only as high as you can without your back muscles kicking in and without pain. Hold for ten seconds.

**Step 6:** Slowly lower yourself back to the starting position using only your arms. Repeat five to ten reps. These can be done daily.

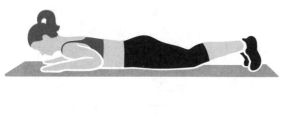

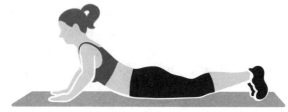

## Stenosis

Severe stenosis can be a serious problem and you may need medical help. But it is also true that often the things we have taught you so far will help quite a lot. Indeed, they may be an answer, so it is worth a try. We do not hold out the promise of an 80 percent success rate with severe stenosis, but the chances of success are substantial and well worth a try. Cases of mild to moderate stenosis typically respond very well to the approaches presented in this book.

The process will seem familiar now. Primarily, it is just a matter of finding (and maintaining) your neutral spine so that the irritation can die down. Once you feel comfortable with neutral spine, start to try walking again. For most people with stenosis, walking for moderate distances can be a problem. Make sure to keep your neutral spine and swing your arms from the shoulders as we talked about earlier. In addition, stop and take breaks and sit down before the pain starts. Eventually try to increase the distance you can go between sitting breaks. With increased fitness and endurance in the core muscles, these times between sitting will get longer and longer. Again, I caution that if you have very severe stenosis, you may be one of the relatively few who need surgery. This is especially true if you have leg symptoms and/or weakness. That said, I have seen countless patients whose MRIs showed moderate to severe stenosis (lateral or central) who were able to get back to a low level of pain and high level of function without surgery. So it is worth a shot.

For many with lateral or central stenosis, bicycling can be a great way to get exercise and relieve the back, because of the forward-bent posture when on a bike. Another solution is to do the following stretch to relieve the discomfort caused by stenosis.

# Stenosis Relief Stretch

This stretch is the knee-to-chest stretch for relief from stenosis. It is pretty simple and often effective.

**Step 1:** Lie on your back.

**Step 2:** Lightly engage your core.

**Step 3:** Slowly bring your knees up toward your chest and grab your knees with your hands, pulling your knees into the chest.

**Step 4:** Hold and breathe for thirty seconds.

**Step 5:** Repeat five to ten times. This can be done throughout the day.

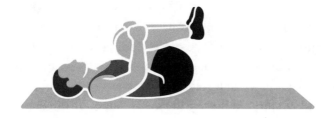

## Scoliosis

If you have scoliosis, it is important to see a good physical therapist to get exercises prescribed for your specific body. One size does not fit all on this one, so we cannot handle it definitively in this book. Your therapist should take into account the degree of curvature you have in your spine and the cause of your scoliosis and prescribe treatment accordingly. For instance, scoliosis caused by a leg length discrepancy will sometimes respond to orthotics. Severe scoliosis might require a brace. There are various exercises and stretches to apply depending on your body. I recommend getting personal help from a skilled therapist while *also* embarking on the protocol presented in this book.

## Pregnancy

Back pain during pregnancy is extremely common. This is because of a host of factors including weight gain, hormonal changes, stress, and lack of sleep. It is a great idea, if you can manage it, to practice all of the advice in this book before you get pregnant and during the early stages of pregnancy. I quite understand that you have a lot on your mind during this period (when I wrote this, Michelle and I were less than a month away from having our first child), but doing these exercises will be a substantial blessing during pregnancy and after. Add it to the list.

Having made that boast, I have to admit that you will likely struggle with back pain to some extent no matter what you do. But the back pain will be a lot less. One of the reasons you get back pain in pregnancy is wonderfully logical: It is the release of the hormone relaxin. It is released into your body to prepare for the birth by causing the ligaments in and around the pelvis to loosen, which is a great idea if you are about to deliver a baby, *but* it also leads to instability in the spine and pelvis, and causes pain. It's a trade-off: It makes the actual delivery easier, but it causes some pain. The more stable and strong you are going into pregnancy, the better your chances of avoiding back pain. But there is this overriding bit of good advice: Regular exercise throughout pregnancy, including many of the exercises in this book (with *light* weight) can be done safely and will help a lot with back pain. Talk to your doctor about which exercises are safe for you and how much weight you can safely lift in each stage of pregnancy. You might want to bring this book to your doctor's appointment for guidance on whether the basic exercises are safe for you.

Is all this worth it, just for the relatively short term of a pregnancy? Yes. First, it is *not* a short term, not if you are in serious back pain. And pregnancy is tough enough without the added burden of back pain. So give the preceding advice some thought. At some point you may have flare-ups of back pain, no matter what you do. At that point, you may want to find a good chiropractor and/or acupuncturist to help you. But find a good one, one who has had lots of experience treating pregnant women. Follow my general advice about finding such professionals. Then ask specific questions about your particular needs and concerns of their office manager when looking to make an appointment.

Okay, that's it for these most demanding "special situations." But I have seen this advice do a lot of good for those in these situations and felt compelled to include it. Again, it is "blended advice": Use the book *and* see a medical or other specialized healer. And it may not give total relief, but there is a good chance that it will help a lot. And that's what we're here for.

## CHAPTER NINETEEN

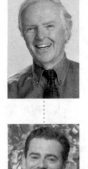

# Congratulations! *And* One Last Assignment

**From Chris and Jeremy**

## From Chris

First of all, congratulations. You have read and (let us hope) absorbed the critical pieces of the James Protocol. That's the big deal; the vast majority of you are now equipped to work on your own to end or radically reduce your back pain, forever. Let me recap: You have learned some moves to help you step out of back pain in the short term so that you can embark on the regimen of exercises and movements that are going to solve the problem in the long term. You have learned how to stop doing the things that got you into this mess in the first place ("stop doing dumb stuff"). You have also learned how to build up endurance and strength in your core. Finally, you have learned how to move in all dimensions while maintaining a neutral spine and bracing your core. That is, you have learned how to move in daily life and do moderate exercise, without hurting your wretched back. Overall, you have learned how to behave differently, and that will make all the difference. Nice work. Very, very nice work. Continue with what you've learned and do the basic exercises every day (hey, it's only for the rest of your life), and there is every reason to hope that most of you will be pain-free (or almost pain-free) from now on. Read the book again, from time to time, be rigorous about doing the exercises, and you're there.

Almost.

There is one more area that we have not covered (a book like this can be only so long) but which we want you to think about. And act on. Note that I said above that you were ready for "moderate exercise." Fine, if that's what you want. But if, as we hope, you decide to move back into the *strenuous* exercise that is such a joy to so many of us—the rugged skiing, the flat-out tennis, the golf, the yoga, and so on—you should think seriously about doing more than we have been able to tell you in the compass of this book. For you—and, frankly, for almost everyone—it makes a lot of sense to adopt a more comprehensive and demanding program of strength training than what we have outlined thus far in order to really strengthen your core and prepare to meet the special demands (for back-pain people) of serious exercise. Others may embark on serious exercise without doing all the core work (maybe), but those with a history of a bad back do so at their peril. Not a good idea.

As I say, we just can't do it here; it is almost another whole book. But we do have two great leads for you and some specific things to focus on (and avoid) as you turn to this phase.

First, the ideas.

For a general, non-back-specific approach to strength training, you cannot do better than to get your hands on the book *Younger Next Year: The Exercise Program*. It is a short but cutting-edge outline of strength training (with exercises by the brilliant Bill Fabrocini) as well as aerobic exercise, which is also key to your long-term recovery. It is not specifically back-oriented, but Bill Fabrocini is very sophisticated about back issues and his general strength-training guidance will serve you well. (Also, I cowrote it, so it is intermittently readable.)

More specifically, Jeremy has just completed a truly remarkable, video-based guide to back pain and exercise (of all kinds) called BackForever.com. As I now know so well, when it comes to back issues Jeremy is an absolute hound for precision, scientific soundness, and detail, and he has worked his tail off to make his subscription video protocol (with some 150 separate videos on absolutely everything) as good and comprehensive as video can be. I have seen 'em, and they're amazing.

Actually, if it were my back, I'd buy the book (it's cheap) and subscribe to BackForever.com (the price of a couple of sessions with a personal trainer). If you do the same, we guarantee you'll end your back pain and live happily ever after. No, we don't, but damn near.

Before we turn you loose, we want to give you some warnings about strength training in general and a couple of specific tips about things to avoid.

## THE BODYBUILDING BLUNDER

The first step for a lot of us, as we turn to strength training, is to "get over" the "bodybuilder" or "muscle isolation" mentality of the 1960s and '70s and beyond. In those decades, the new exercise machines—Nautilus and others—were all in vogue, as was the focus on bodybuilding, thanks in significant part to Arnold Schwarzenegger and the movie *Pumping Iron*. The idea was to build big biceps ("guns"), huge quads, and whatnot. And to become strong. Then I guess you head down to the beach so Gidget and the *Baywatch* babes could swarm around. And the way you built those guns and whatnot, mostly, was with the nifty new weightlifting machines, especially the Nautilus gadgets. The ostensible genius of the Nautilus machines was that they gave constant stress across the full range of a rep. True, too, and a good idea. But the *real* appeal of the machines, I bet, was that in some curious way they made weightlifting "easy." You still had to hoist heavy weights and grunt and sweat and stuff. *But* the machines did a lot of the hardest and most subtle work. *They took all the* balance *out of strength training. And most of the coordination.* Which permitted you to do what bodybuilders wanted to do then which was to *isolate* and grow the big muscles: the quads, your pecs, your biceps, and so on. It was much easier to do all that if you did not have to bother with the pesky business of balancing and stabilizing yourself.

In the normal course of weight training (when you were not using strength machines), stability (and coordination) was mostly the work of little support muscles and groups of muscles surrounding the big muscles. The machines did most of that for you. Which was nice. Except for this: The little guys—the support muscles—atrophied or died. Which was dangerous and dumb.

Because our body is designed to work—virtually all the time—on a fully integrated, whole-body basis. And that is impossible without the help of the little guys. Athletic movements (and most real-life movements) do not use isolated muscles; they use the whole shebang. Movement and exercise is orchestral, not a series of solos. Every lift in the real world is a *whole-body* affair. Isolating the big boys while letting the little guys go to hell was an absolutely awful idea. Bill Fabrocini (one of the great leaders in the whole-body training field and coauthor of two Younger Next Year books on the subject) sees hundreds of well-intentioned, serious people now in their sixties and seventies who have been "muscle isolation" weightlifters all their lives. They have huge muscles and can hoist great weight with them. But for the activities of daily life or normal exercise, they are weak as kittens. They are wretched athletes (if they can move at all). And often *their backs and necks are aching ruins*. Because the little muscles, which are key to whole-body movement, have gone to hell and their bodies are agonizingly out of alignment. It is possible to save these poor souls but it takes forever. Unsurprisingly, it is mostly a matter of teaching them to get over the machines and the muscle isolation model and learn whole-body, integrated workouts. Mostly you use your own body weight in integrated exercises, without machines. (Note: You do not have to give up machines completely; they can be a useful supplement to a whole-body regimen, if used properly.)

Did that help? I hope so. Because it is important to grasp the significance of integrated, whole-body strength training. It is only integrated, whole-body movement that is going to build the kind of strength and movement patterns that are going to enable you to return to those higher risk activities. And make no mistake: You are almost certainly going to have to develop a much stronger core if it is going to be able to do its great job in protecting your back for serious exercise.

## From Jeremy

Let me expand upon the muscle isolation theme a bit. Often it may be necessary to isolate muscles when deficiencies are present in those particular muscles, to reestablish strength and balance within the body so that a full-body exercise can be performed properly. But, after these rehabilitative goals are accomplished, integrated movement using the core for stability while incorporating balance is essential. With most machines, you are sitting there, exerting maximum force across *one joint*—your elbow, say—while the machine does all the stabilizing and balancing. That puts dangerous amounts of load across that joint. Bodybuilding focuses on developing muscle hypertrophy, meaning an increase in muscle mass. A specific muscle or set of muscles is isolated with a machine and moved against resistance until that muscle gets big. Various muscles throughout the body are put through this process individually to achieve a certain look, with no thought given to linking the muscles together to mimic the movements of sport or daily activities. This does nothing to train the muscles and muscle systems to *move* . . . to work together for maximum efficiency and minimum joint damage. As we age, it is crucial to challenge the systems in our bodies that maintain balance and stability. As the saying goes, use it or lose it.

Instead of bodybuilding, we want you to think of training *muscle systems and movements*. A maxim I hear Bill say all the time that is common in the profession is "*Train movement, not muscles*," and he's absolutely right. Your goal in the gym is to build up the systems of muscles that support the movements of daily life, work, and sport, not to build "guns" for the beach.

You also need to get out of the mind-set that to work your core you must be doing core-specific exercises. It doesn't work that way. All whole-body exercises are core exercises. The core muscles are designed to *stop* movement, not produce movement. Think about that for a minute. The core muscles are there to stop your spine and torso from moving while loads are applied through the arms and legs. Their primary function isn't so much to move the torso as to keep it still. For example, if you are standing on your own two feet with nothing to lean against and pull a cable that has resistance, it is your core that is keeping your body from twisting and becoming off balance when you pull the cable.

The stronger the resistance on the cable, the stronger your core has to be to resist that resistance. Juxtapose this with sitting on a "seated row" machine, where your chest is against a pad and you pull enormous amounts of weight, straining against the pad to keep your body in place, and you get the picture.

## DETAILS

Just as in your daily exercises laid out in painstaking detail in this book thus far, the specific little details matter in strength training with weights, too. In fact, the stakes are higher because the load is higher and there is far less room for error. Regarding weight training, your goals dictate the degree of risk you are willing to assume. All weight training requires you to assume some degree of risk. If your goal is to get back to being an NBA center, that risk is pretty high because we are going to subject you to enormous loads in somewhat dangerous positions, but it's worth it if you need to get back to your multimillion-dollar-a-year job. If your goal is to get back to being a grandma who can safely pick up her grandchild, the risk is much lower. And if your goal is to get back to recreational golf a few times a week, your risk is somewhere in the middle. It is for these reasons and because of the complexity of the movements we are discussing that presenting a one-size-fits-all strength-training regimen in this book is nearly impossible. Therefore we decided that rather than present you with an inferior product, we would give you an overview of the general information here and present you with some options to further your interests in a much more individualized way.

As you know, Chris and I are both huge fans of Bill Fabrocini's warm-ups and exercises in *Younger Next Year: The Exercise Program*. They provide a superb foundation for general strength training. If you want a more customized workout tailored to the protection and strengthening of your back check out my BackForever.com online membership program with streaming videos and other content referred to in the Appendix. It was my goal to make it the *definitive, visual guide* in this area.

Another option of course is to hire a personal trainer until you get comfortable with the do's and don'ts of strength training. A great personal trainer can be a huge help. But be warned, personal trainers vary wildly in skill level and knowledge. It can be very difficult to find a good one. Asking potential trainers if they are familiar with the concepts we talk about in this book is a good starting point. Also ask how much experience they have with working with clients with back pain. Ask them for referrals and interview those people if possible. Chris and I hope to solve the problem of finding a good trainer by creating a certification program down the road. Depending on where you live, expect to pay anywhere from $75 to $200 per hour for a great personal trainer.

## From Chris and Jeremy

Finally, we also want to drive home the point about strength exercises that are bad for you. There are a few that you just shouldn't be doing. Even though we don't have room to show you the things you *should* do instead, we wanted to give you a sharp warning about the things you should not do. We include these "bad exercises" here so you don't hurt yourself.

### BEHIND THE HEAD LAT PULLDOWNS

This bad boy places the shoulder in a vulnerable position that can lead to injury of the rotator cuff and shoulder joint. It also puts enormous strain on the cervical spine (neck) because of the forward head position. Instead try lat pulldowns to the chest or pull-ups (if you are obscenely strong). We're not going to get into how to do stuff right here, but here's a tiny tip: When you do *front* lat pulldowns, do them standing, not sitting. You do more to strengthen the core and glutes. Just saying....

## SMITH SQUATS ARE A BUM IDEA FOR MANY

Smith exercise machines were designed to help people squat with a heavy load while minimizing the risk of the lifter collapsing due to a built-in catch mechanism. That part makes sense. But there's a problem: The machine guides the bar in one plane of motion, which won't allow most people to do a functional squat on it. The squat is a very complicated, important, and

**Lat pull down alternative**

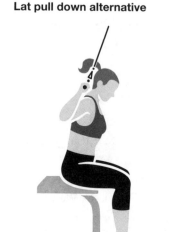

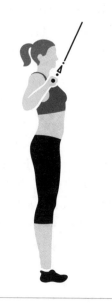

**BAD**

GOOD

*personal* exercise for back health (see Chapter 13 to get it right). By "personal" I mean that no two bodies are the same and no two sets of (good) squats are the same. The Smith machine doesn't allow for that. Its "one-size-fits-all" approach can create bad squats for many people, which can lead to knee, hip, and back problems down the road. I'd skip it.

### SIT-UPS

We hit this before, but it's so important we want to mention it again. If you were to set out to design an exercise to ruin lumbar discs you would be hard-pressed to design one more effective at that task than the full "army sit-up." Why? The discs in your low back are damaged by repetitive flexion, aka

**Smith squat alternative**

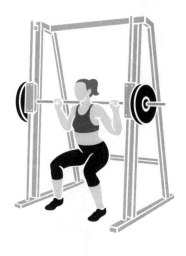

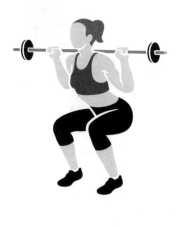

**BAD**                     GOOD

## Sit-up alternative

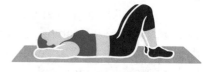

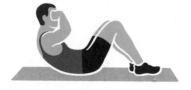

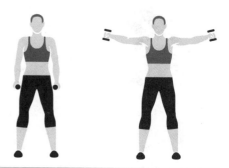

**BAD**

**GOOD**

## Shrug alternative

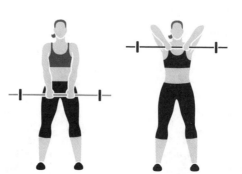

**BAD**

**GOOD**

forward bending and twisting. Sit-ups and especially sit-ups with rotation at the end (where you rotate to touch your right elbow to your left knee) reproduce these damaging movements exactly. Instead, do the crunches and planks in the daily routine we have given you. Those will be more than adequate to build the core and back strength you need and in a much safer way.

### SHRUGS

This exercise places the shoulder into internal rotation, putting the supraspinatus and its tendon at serious risk of injury over time. It also places a lot of stress on the cervical spine. Instead, do "full can," as shown in the illustration. Pick two relatively light dumbbells to start. Grip one in each hand with hands by your sides. Stand with good posture. Slowly lift the weights up to shoulder level, with your arms coming up at a 45-degree angle from the front and sides of your body (not straight to the side, or straight to the front, but in between). Do ten to twelve repetitions. As with all exercises that involve the arms and shoulders, make sure your shoulder blades stay down and back throughout the movement, especially when lifting upward.

Okay. We have given you some dire warnings and some general guidance to doing strength training correctly. Now, if you want to get back into some of these higher-risk, higher-intensity athletic and other activities, have a look at Jeremy's BackForever.com website and go for it!

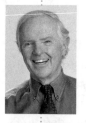

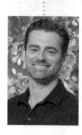

**CHAPTER TWENTY**

# The Sacrum
# and Coccyx

**From Chris and Jeremy**

## From Chris

The sacrum is the last section of the spine, the vestigial collection of vertebrae that are welded into one solid piece, down at the bottom. And the coccyx is the tippety-tip of the sacrum, the last bit of bone at the end of that long chain, which has been such a torment to you for so long.

And this is the end of the book. The end of the long chain of chapters that we hope—with all our hearts—will deliver you from such torment forever. From now on, it's up to you. Go back through the book, do the exercises, and *change your behavior* the way you know you should. Up to you now.

May I say, here at the end, that putting this book together has been great fun for Jeremy and me. It has taken more than a year, and it has been a ton of work. We hope it reads as if it were easy as pie, but it wasn't. We worked like crazy to make it *seem* easy—and to make it truly accurate without driving you crazy. Don't know how well we did on that, but we sure did try. And it was fun for a couple of reasons. First, from my point of view, Jeremy is awfully good company. He is deadly serious about his profession but he loves to laugh, too. And, God bless us, we think we're funny. That helped a lot. On a slightly more serious note, learning all the stuff I had to learn about the back this past year was fascinating and a privilege. Interesting piece of machinery, the back, and Jeremy could not have been a better guide.

Finally, both of us are true believers in this "revolution" I mentioned up front, and that is a tremendous help. The whole time we were digging away at this boring detail or that, we had the agreeable conviction that we were not just ink-stained wretches, noses to the page. We were centurions in the great war against cruel, needless pain. That helped a lot, too.

But the whole business won't be satisfying to us if it doesn't work, for you. And that takes me back to my one great worry, the one I mentioned before.

I worry that we leave so much of this up to you, when we know that Americans just aren't used to that. Americans are used to going to the magician/doctor. He has a look around, maybe does an MRI. And then hands us a prescription, or gives us a shot. Or sends us to his pal the back surgeon, who does some clever thing to make us all better. As we've said again and again, that's not going to work here. You have to do it yourself— you have to do the exercise, make the changes. But the great question is, will you find the resolve to make it happen? Jeremy says he's sure you will, because he knows your pain. He knows just how deep and sharp your motivation is. I hope he's right.

What we are urging is not really that hard; it is mostly just unfamiliar. And you surely have the resources and motivation to make it happen. I know you're smart enough; you just read this darned book, after all. I know you are disciplined enough; you've been going to work all these years. And I know you care, because I know about your pain. Now just take those three things and reorient them a little. And save your life. Then spread the word and save your family, save the country. Get the ogre out of all our lives. It can and should be done.

## From Jeremy

I can't agree more with Chris's words. He and I had such a great time writing this book, and we are both deeply optimistic about what it can do for you. As you well know by now, I am not the "word guy"; that's Chris. So I will be uncharacteristically brief and just say I have seen this protocol work a thousand times in my practice. Now I want to see it work a million times, perhaps more than that, with this book. As we mentioned at the beginning, we want a revolution in back care in this country. Starting with you. We want to take this scourge out of all our lives.

# JEREMY'S RULES

## 1
Stop doing dumb stuff.

## 2
Be still so you can heal.

## 3
Brace yourself.

## 4
Commit to your core.

## 5
Use the power in your posterior.

## 6
Crawl before you walk. Walk before you run.

## 7
Stand tall for the long haul.

# Appendix

## The "Cheat Sheet"

W e threw a lot at you in this book. In time, it will seem like second nature. When you get to that point, it may still be useful to have a simple guide to remind you where you are, what to do next, and so on. To that end, I give you this "cheat sheet" to summarize all the exercises we have told you to do and to tell you when to do them. Here is your daily and weekly plan.

I strongly encourage you to read this book a few times a year. Trust me, you are trying to change lifelong habits and it's very easy to default back to the old ways. Come back to the book and think through each exercise every so often. Avoid the trap of falling into those same bad habits that got you here in the first place. The book is the key to taking your life back and leaving the anxiety, stress, and pain of back problems in the past. In between readings of the book, there's this Exercise Cheat Sheet.

## Basic Core Exercises

These exercises (see Chapter 10) should be done every day, and are best done in the morning after being out of bed for thirty minutes or so. Remember to do progressions or regressions as needed for each. Move on to the next progression of a particular exercise when and if you feel ready. Start with one circuit and work your way up to two full circuits in time, and make that your daily habit. In time, this will take you ten to fifteen minutes.

1. Slow March with Neutral Spine with Shoulder Flexion

2. The Bridge

3. Crunch and Plank

4. Dynamic Hamstring Stretch

5. Side Plank

6. Cat/Camel Mobilization

7. "Bird Dog," or Opposite Arm/Leg Extension

## Glute Strengthening Routine

Do these exercises three times a week on nonconsecutive days in addition to your core routine. Start with two sets and work your way up to three in time. This will likely add an additional ten minutes or so on those three days a week that you do these.

1. Hip Circles (Chapter 17) Do these first!

2. Clamshell (Chapter 13)

3. Quadruped Hip Extension (Chapter 10)

4. Split Squat (Chapter 13)

5. Squat (Chapter 13)

## Trigger Point Release

Do this as needed. If you got noticeable improvement in back, hip, or leg pain after mastering this, do it prior to your glute workouts until it is no longer needed.

## Stretches

Follow up your glute routine with the following stretches from Chapter 17.

**This will take three to four minutes.**

1. Hamstring Stretch

2. Glute Stretch

3. Piriformis Stretch

4. Psoas Stretch

---

**THE BACKFOREVER VIDEOS**

For those of you who want to safely return to more demanding activities like weightlifting, skiing, golf, tennis, Pilates, yoga, etc., we invite you to become members of BackForever.com, where you will find hundreds of hours of detailed video instruction on these subjects. Visit BackForever.com to learn more. Enter this promo code to receive two free weeks of membership: YNYTRIAL.

# Acknowledgments

Thanks to Jeremy, first of all, for being such a joy to work with. Coauthorship is supposed to be hard. For me—especially in this book—it has been a joy. We worked mighty hard, but we laughed a lot too.

Jeremy and I have been blessed—and we know it—to have a superb editor in a smart, kind, diplomatic, literate Bruce Tracy at Workman. (That is a shortened list of attributes; Bruce was terrific. And he really got down into the weeds as well as the big picture. As good as they get.) And, as always, thanks to the wise and kind Suzie Bolotin, editor of the Younger Next Year® books and Uber-editor of this one. Heaven!

Last, thanks to Bill Fabrocini, just about the smartest and most effective guy Jeremy and I know in the broad world of physical therapy and serious training. And about as nice a human being as I have ever met. Deep thanks, Bill.

—*C. C.*

I'd like to thank all of the people who have helped me become the clinician I am today. I'd like to thank Clinton Phillips, Michael Fox, Tim Powersmith, and Bill Fabrocini for their friendship, guidance, and the opportunities they have given me. Back pain has been one of the most misunderstood afflictions in modern society. Many of the concepts in this book are the result of the research and teaching of a handful of dedicated and pioneering individuals. There are many, but I would like to give special mention to Vladimir Janda, MD; David Simons, MD; Janet Travell, MD; Nikolai Bogduk, MD, PhD; and Stuart McGill, PhD. This book wouldn't have been possible without your accomplishments.

—*J. J.*

# About the Authors

**Chris Crowley,** a retired litigation partner at Davis Polk & Wardwell in New York, is the coauthor, with Henry S. Lodge, MD, of the Younger Next Year books and, with Jen Sacheck, PhD, of *Thinner This Year*. In his eighties he is living the life, hard: skiing the black diamonds in the Rockies, doing fifty-mile bike loops, rowing his single scull, and giving lectures all over the country as well as finishing a novel. He lives with his wife, Hilary, in New York City and Lakeville, Connecticut.

**Jeremy James, DC, CSCS,** is founder of Backforever.com and for many years directed a successful destination clinic for chronic back-pain sufferers. He became a Doctor of Chiropractic (instead of going into traditional medicine like almost everyone else in his family) because of his own struggles with sports-induced back pain as a young athlete, and developed his behavioral/whole-body method while working with serious athletes for over a decade. He lives with his wife and son in Aspen, Colorado.

Chris Crowley is a regular keynote speaker all over the world on Younger Next Year® and related topics. To hire Chris to speak, contact him at Chris@Youngernextyear.com.

# Index

## A

abdominal muscles, 39

## B

back muscles, 38–39
"Bicycles" on Your Side, 219
Bird Dog, 126–32
Bridge, 103–107
   One-Leg Bridge, 105–7
bulging disc, 28, 31, 41–42
   patient stories, 56–57, 60, 78
   suggestions for relief, 220
burst disc. *See* herniated disc

## C

Cat/Camel Mobilization, 124–25
chiropractor, finding a, 202–4
Clamshell, 150–53
   with Resistance, 153–54
core, 12–13
   engaging your core, 92–93
   tightening, 90–91
creep, 67–70
Crunch, 108–10

## D

driving posture, 200

## E

engaging your core, 92–93
exercises to avoid, 233–37

## F

fascia connective tissue, 40
foraminal canal and stenosis,
   44–46, 48, 52
Full-Body Rotation, 185–86

## G

Getting Out of a Chair, 195–96
Getting Up off the Floor, 197–98
gluteus
   finding trigger points, 170–72
   Glute Stretch, 210
   gluteal muscles, 148–50
   releasing trigger points, 173–74

## H

hamstring
   Dynamic Hamstring Stretch,
      115–16
   Hamstring Stretch, 209
herniated disc, 2, 41–42, 57
Hip Circles, 207
hip extensions
   quadruped, 129–30, 154–55
   standing, 155–57
hip-hinge
   with Neutral Spine, 182–84
   Torso Rotation with Squat,
      187–89
hypermobile sacroiliac (SI) joint
   pain, 215–16

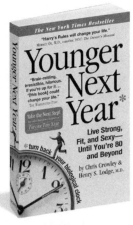
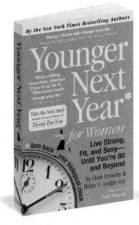
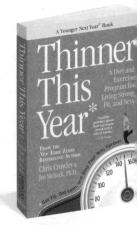
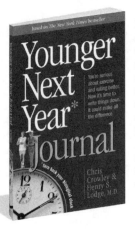
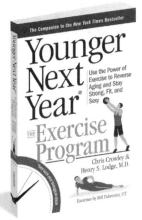
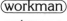